Vagus Nerve, Vagal Tone & Polyvagal Theory

Activate Your Natural Healing Power to Reduce Depression, Anxiety and Stress

Erika Newton

Table of Contents

The Polyvagal Theory

Erika Newton

Introduction

Customarily the autonomic nervous system was perceived for its guideline of the different instinctive "programmed" capacities, for example, absorption, breath, sex drive, propagation, and so on. The old model of pressure or unwinding depended on perceiving just two circuits—the sympathetic and the parasympathetic. In the old model, the sympathetic nervous system was viewed as dynamic in stress reaction to dangers and risk. The parasympathetic nervous system, on the other hand, communicated in the unwinding reaction and was related to the capacity of the vagus nerve. This more established, all-around acknowledged model of the autonomic nervous system expected that there is a solitary vagus nerve, and it didn't assess the way that there are really two very unique neural pathways that are both called "vagus."

The Polyvagal Theory starts by perceiving that the vagus nerve has two separate branches—two discrete, particular vagal nerves that begin in two unique areas. We get a progressively exact portrayal of the operations of the autonomic nervous system. The autonomic nervous system comprises three neural circuits: the ventral branch of the vagus nerve (positive states of unwinding and social engagement), the spinal sympathetic chain (battle or flight), and the dorsal branch of the vagus nerve (slowdown, shutdown, and burdensome conduct). These three circuits direct our substantial capacities so as to assist our bodies with homeostasis.

The Polyvagal Theory likewise displays another measurement to our comprehension of the autonomic nervous system. The autonomic nervous system not just controls the capacity of our inward organs; these three circuits additionally identify with our emotional states, which thusly drive our conduct. Individuals who give massages know for a fact that one individual's body may be excessively tight, another may be excessively delicate, and a third can feel "perfect." Usually, when specialists are prepared to give a massage, they figure out how to discharge pressure in a strained muscle. Notwithstanding, this methodology doesn't take a shot at a body that needs adequate tone.

Movement bolstered by the spinal sympathetic chain empowers us to battle so as to meet danger head-on or flee to maintain a strategic distance from it. This is because hard, tense muscles allow us to move the whole body more rapidly. Worse hypertension is additionally expected to get the flow of blood into muscles that are strained and hard.

Low levels of muscle tonus are discovered when the dorsal vagal circuit is actuated when there is no compelling reason to tense the muscles to battle or escape (or, at times of outrageous threat, when the body's endurance reaction is too close down). Low blood pressure is adequate to get the blood into delicate, limp muscles. In its outrageous structure, this low blood pressure may make individuals lose cognizance and swoon. The restorative term for this is "syncope." Normal blood pressure is suitable for neither tense nor limp muscles. In states of social engagement, there is commonly no risk or threat in our condition or body. Our nervous system activates this reality, so we don't need to do anything; we can genuinely unwind and appreciate being with others. As far as the Polyvagal Theory, we can

7

be immobilized, unafraid, outraged, or feel burdensome when we are in a condition of social engagement. Our blood pressure, blood sugar, and temperature are generally typical. We can stay composed yet wakeful and alert.

A handshake gives us a decent sign of the condition of someone else's autonomic nervous system. An excessively tight body, as a rule, results from an incessant condition of action in the spinal sympathetic chain, where the whole solid system is ceaselessly arranged to battle or escape. Such an individual typically has an excessively compelling handshake, pressing more earnestly than would normally be appropriate. The inverse is valid for somebody lacking strong tonus—generally an indication of over-movement in the dorsal vagal circuit. This individual, by and large, has a limp, moist, and, every now and then, chilly handshake. In the event that our handshake is perfect, it is the ventral branch of the vagus nerve that is transcendent. We may have a few pressures in individual muscles. However, the strained muscles loosen up rapidly, and a massage specialist will see that our body likewise feels right. The tonus of the muscles is just one of numerous approaches to screening the condition of the body's nervous system.

HOMEOSTASIS AND THE ANS

The neural circuits controlling the nerves managing instinctive organ capacity can be contrasted with an indoor regulator connected to both a warmer and a forced-air system. At the point when the indoor regulator enlists that the air is excessively chilly, it turns on the warmer, and if the air is excessively warm, it turns into a real-time conditioner. Warm-blooded creatures comparably need to keep up internal heat level within upper and lower limits, and their tactile nerves give criticism about internal heat level to their "indoor regulator."

Standards of conduct, just as physiological capacities, help the body to direct temperature. For instance, if we are cold, we can move around to create heat through the action of our muscles, or we can put on more garments to protect ourselves and reduce the loss of body heat. The blood vessels of the skin choke to save heat. When we are freezing, our bodies begin to shudder wildly, creating heat from the activity of the muscles. At the point when we are warm, we rest or sit still so as to diminish strong movement and, in this way, stay away from further overheating. The blood vessels enlarge, allowing more warmth to arrive at the skin surface, where it very well may be scattered. We take off layers of apparel, and we sweat; when our perspiration vanishes, it cools the body. At the point when individuals are irate, we now and then state that they are "angry as a mad bull." We may reprove them to "cool it." When individuals don't care for something, they may pull back, and we state that they are "cool" to it. We consider approaches to "warm them up" to the thought. Both warmth and coolness are detected as impressions of emotional states.

The three parts of the autonomic nervous system cooperate to control the action of the organs, realize homeostasis, and assist us with suitably meeting ecological circumstances and equalization conditions inside the body. We can likewise apply the model of the Polyvagal Theory to issues and findings in numerous physiological territories, for example, assimilation or proliferation, which we may somehow or another consider to be physical issues outside our ability to control or impact. For instance, a developing collection of logical research utilizes pulse changeability (HRV) to gauge ventral vagal movement by measuring an unconstrained beat in pulse known as respiratory sinus arrhythmia. These examinations locate that low degrees of ventral vagal action are connected to a wide scope of medical problems, for example, weight, hypertension, heart variances, and so on. There are likewise a few hypotheses that HRV is a possibly valuable estimation to help anticipate the beginning of a disease, malignant growth metastasis, or the reasonable mortality of individuals with diseases.

The Five States of the Autonomic Nervous System

BIOBEHAVIOR: THE INTERACTION OF BEHAVIOR AND BIOLOGICAL PROCESSES

In contrast to the old model of the autonomic nervous system, which concentrated only on its guideline of the capacity of the instinctive organs, the new model of the autonomic nervous system incorporates three particular neural pathways, as discussed above, and relates every one of these three neural circuits with a passionate state, which drives our conduct. Notwithstanding these three states, we have two half and half expresses, every one of which consolidates two of the individual circuits, for an aggregate of five potential states of our autonomic nervous system. One half and half state bolster the experience of closeness: the dorsal vagus is locked in to hinder our physical movement, simultaneously as the ventral vagus permits a sentiment of wellbeing with someone else. This is talked about in further detail beneath.

The subsequent half and half state communicate in a benevolent challenge. We may contend energetically to win in sports or games, yet this happens inside a system of security and rules to which the entirety of the rivals have concurred ahead of time. In this cross breed expression, the battle or flight reaction of spinal thoughtful chain initiation is joined with the sentiments of wellbeing related to the action of the ventral vagus branch.

THE THREE NEURAL PATHWAYS OF THE ANS

The first of the autonomic nervous system's neural pathways is the social commitment nervous system. It includes action in the ventral branch of the vagus nerve (CN X) and four other cranial nerves (CN V, VII, IX, and XI). Movement in this circuit has a quieting, relieving impact and advances rest and compensation. The ventral branch of the vagus nerve identifies with positive feelings of bliss, fulfillment, and love. When it comes to conduct, it communicates in positive social exercises with companions and friends, and family. The condition of social commitment bolsters social practices in which we back up and offer help to other individuals. Collaboration with others typically improves our odds for endurance—we talk together, sing together, move together, share a supper, coordinate to finish a task, instruct and sustain youngsters, and so on.

The second of the ANS's neural pathways is the spinal thoughtful chain, which is enacted when our endurance is undermined. In the event that we assemble our body with this reaction, we can attempt to assist us with reacting to the risk. This condition of "assembly with dread" emerges when we are not protected or don't have a sense of security. Condition of "activation with dread" emerges when we are not sheltered or don't have a sense of security. The spinal thoughtful chain identifies with feelings of outrage or dread, which can convey

11

what needs to be in practice, for example, battling to defeat the danger or escaping to keep away from an undermining circumstance.

The third neural pathway is the dorsal branch of the vagus nerve. This pathway is actuated when we face a staggering power and up-and-coming annihilation. When there is no reason for battling or fleeing, we moderate what assets we have—we immobilize. Actuation of this pathway cultivates sentiments of vulnerability, misery, and lack of care showing in withdrawal and shutdown. This state can be portrayed as "immobilization with dread." When people or different well-evolved creatures are looked at with apparently inescapable human threat, demise, or devastation, the dorsal branch of our vagus nerve is initiated. An abrupt or outrageous flood of dorsal vagal action can offer ascent to a condition of stun or shutdown. Among different reactions, the solid system loses its tonus, and the pulse drops. We may black out or go into a condition of stun (syncope).

Natural life documentaries on the African fields have caught the accompanying scene. A lion pursues and catches a baby antelope and takes it up in its forceful jaws. The baby antelope had been in a condition of spinal thoughtful chain action when it was undermined and fled. Presently, confronting fast approaching passing, it goes into stun and shutdown: it swoons, and its body goes limp. Lions are not by and large foragers. On the off chance that a lion all of a sudden develops faculties that tell it that its prey has gotten dormant, it might open its jaws, drop the prey, and move away. Exactly when the lion is going to shake the baby antelope to break its neck or dive into its tissue, the limp muscles neglect to give the typical obstruction. Maybe the antelope's shutdown reaction is sufficient to invalidate the lion's executioner impulse. The lion discharges its grasp, the baby antelope tumbles to the ground, and the lion moves away.

A few moments after the lion leaves, the baby antelope stands up, shakes it off, and returns to its mom. It, at that point, resumes touching as though nothing has occurred. The baby antelope is prepared to confront the following to test its endurance because of its lifesaving shutdown reaction. This represents the versatile endurance estimation of the dorsal-branch immobilization reaction in circumstances of outrageous risk. We see another case of how the dorsal branch of the vagus nerve can encourage a fruitful barrier: A porcupine, confronting peril from a predator, pulls back by folding up into a ball. Its sharp plumes fiber out-ward, making it next to impossible for the predator to effectively nibble it.

The Two-Hybrid Circuits

Notwithstanding these three circuits of the autonomic nervous system, there are two hybrid states comprised of various mixes of two of the three neural circuits. The fourth state is a hybrid that supports benevolent challenge, or "preparation unafraid," which is there for when we take part in aggressive games. This state joins the impacts of two neural circuits: enactment of the spinal thoughtful chain enables us to assemble ourselves to accomplish our best execution. Actuation of the social commitment circuit keeps things cordial, so we can play securely inside the guidelines and abstain from harming one another.

In sports, we can contend energetically to win. The two groups consent to observe the guidelines and remain within limits to protect everything. All things considered, it is just a game. There are numerous different instances of activating bravery. Young doggies from a similar litter always play with one another as though they were battling. They snarl and chomp each other for a considerable length of time.

The fifth state is additionally a hybrid of two neural circuits. Action in the dorsal part of the vagus nerve, when joined with that of the ventral part of the vagus nerve, underpins sentiments of closeness and private conduct. This state, which we could call "immobilization unafraid," is described as a quiet that confides in sentiments, permitting us, for instance, to lie still and nestle with a friend or family member.

NOTES

Chapter 1:

The Evolution of Polyvagal Theory

A t the point when I began my logical profession, I was interested in the plausibility of utilizing physiological measures to comprehend the mental conditions of others. In the late 1960s, when I was in graduate school, I had the vision that observing a physiological state would be a useful manual for the advisor during clinical communication. This vision is still a piece of my inquire about motivation. I am as yet taking a shot at building up a polyvagal screen, which will give input progressively to clinicians of the dynamic interchange between the three neural circuits depicted in the polyvagal theory.

During the 1960s, the developments and models relating physiology to conduct were constrained. Prevailing in human and psychophysiological writing was a build of excitement. The characterizing highlights of excitement were dubious. In any case, psychophysiologists expected that the thoughtful apprehensive framework intervened arousal. Early psychophysiologists, for example, Chester Darrow, proposed coherence between cortical initiation estimated through electroencephalography (EEG), what's more, thoughtful excitement estimated by the galvanic skin obstruction reaction on the hands. This perspective on a fringe marker of mind forms was reliable with Pavlov's utilization of autonomic measures in his traditional molding tests. For Pavlov, the "traditionally" molded autonomic reactions were lists of changes in cerebrum circuits. Excitement is as yet utilized in the rest of the research to portray cortical enactment and inquire about the trickery in which customary polygraphs are utilized. The particular physiological and neurophysiological components of basic excitement are regularly connected with the thoughtful sensory system and the hypothalamic-pituitary-adrenal (HPA) hub. An induced association between the thoughtful sensory system and the HPA pivot has brought about comparative research strategies being utilized to think about both excitement and stress. This thoughtful, driven view has been converted into the mainstream press and open cognizance as an antique that a restricted measure of pressure is "great," and an excess of stress is "terrible." But what were the limits of pressure important for wellbeing or disease? What's more, reliable with this sympathetic-centric view, we as a whole were instructed that the stress-related thoughtful excitation had transformative causes in mammalian fight or flight practices. In this way, we were instructed that the expanded thoughtful tone of oddity and threat was an impression of our developmental history.

The polyvagal theory is a comprehension of the reiteration of our developmental history. For well-evolved creatures, the developmental history is really called phylogeny, which deals with the sensory systems (or their highlights) that we've acquired from our precursors. For this situation, the predecessors are reptiles, land, and water proficient, furthermore, fish. As vertebrates, we have acquired a lot of circuits. As these circuits transform, they brought about utilitarian neuro-stages for a large number of the practices we as people express. One thing we have overlooked or didn't comprehend until the polyvagal theory empowered us to have the reconceptualization was our extraordinary progress from reptiles to warm-blooded animals. In that progress from old reptiles to even the crude warm-blooded animals, certain things happened. Those things are tied in with empowering co-guideline in a sense, empowering one well-evolved creature to help direct the physiological condition of another well-evolved creature. That required prompting, or the social commitment, of another with signals of wellbeing and signs of security to empower two of the species to be agreeable in one another's essence.

The entire history of warm-blooded creatures is tied in with being agreeable within sight of another proper warm-blooded animal. It's truly what gets disturbed with injury. At the point when an injury happens, individuals are never again ready to cohabitate with another, since regularly the injury has been delivered by another person and their sensory system presently doesn't welcome the other individual into their quality. The polyvagal model truly has three polyvagal states, including the crudest framework that we've acquired, which is imparted to for all intents and purposes all vertebrates. It returns to the ligament that fish have, which is identified with the capacity to immobilize with dread and utilize fixed status as a guard framework. This becomes one of the basic focuses – that is, people who have gone into a breakdown or a demise faking have changed on the grounds that they've obtained access to this extremely old knowledge. Hereditarily, the following stage that developed was the assembly framework, which we as a whole know as battle flight. In any case, battle flight likewise has certain magnificent points of interest, since as long as we continue moving, we're not going to be defenseless against closed down or breakdown. You see those side effects in numerous individuals who have injury chronicles.

Being in a physiological condition of battle flight isn't awesome for one's body. It prompts ailments. It's additionally shocking for social communications since we need to sign others to, as it were, remain quiet, co-control, and offer encounters. We could utilize the term between abstract encounters. We need to share contemplations and thoughts and all things considered to be available with another. With the appearance of warm-blooded animals, a more up-to-date circuit went ahead, and this is what we're naming either the ventral vagal circuit or the social commitment framework. The social commitment framework was really connecting the neuro-guideline of all the muscles, the strident muscles that control the face and head – including the muscles of vocalization, the muscles of tuning in, the muscles of prompting in the face, also, the muscles of how we articulate the prosodic highlights in our voice with the vagal guideline of the heart.

We fundamentally are continually wearing our face on our heart, and we're passing on our physiological state in our voice. We are identifying the physiological condition of others through their voices and with their countenances. When we watch somebody, we get signals from the speaker's face, tuning in to their voice and choosing if this is an agreeable individual to listen to. Or on the other hand, whether or not I should consider the words or if it would be a good idea for me to consider the sentiments that the words pass on. So the social commitment framework is truly what makes people human or really makes a warm-blooded creature's vertebrate.

The social commitment framework is this superb capacity to pass on to another what our physiological state is. What the polyvagal theory assembles is the view that these circuits are progressive. Progressive implies that more up-to-date circuits have the ability to restrain the more seasoned ones. This means social commitment can down-manage battle flight and can quiet us down similarly as a battle flight can keep us out of closing down. There are three levels, and everyone represses the more crude framework underneath it. The word that was utilized to portray this is a word called "disintegration," which originates from researcher John Hughlings Jackson, who was exceptionally intrigued by cerebrum forms and in this hindrance of mind circuits, with the goal that they become more crude and receptive when we have cerebrum harm or ailment. So the autonomic sensory system works a similar way. Our most up-to-date circuit quiets us; our more seasoned circuits can be utilized for safeguard.

What enables social commitment to happen while the guarded systems of fight-flight are being debilitated? Stephen utilizes the expression "include identifiers" that essentially expect that our sensory system developed to identify includes in the other, to assist us with distinguishing wellbeing. So those component finders are a piece of the build he calls "neuroception." You can't talk about the social commitment framework without discussing neuroception. Neuroception is the instrument through which our sensory system identifies wellbeing and afterward empowers the social commitment framework to work. It distinguishes this without mindfulness. It is a unique framework since it isn't the subjective mindfulness we are in a safe environment.

Our sensory system is identifying the degree of security; at that point, the physiology reacts. One can be extremely mindful of their physiology. Much like setting off to an address, we go in, and we state, "Well, the words sound great or if nothing else if I somehow managed to understand it, it would be great, however you know, there is something in particular about that individual that I don't generally feel great with." Everyone has had those issues. It is difficult to mark; however, we feel awkward; perhaps it's an absence of prosody in that individual's voice, the absence of commitment. We could state it is the absence of being extremely delicate or then again having the feeling that the other is being a substantial individual. It's actually that the words are there, yet the emotions underneath the words may not be. That is the thing that our bodies are reacting to. We react more significantly to the lessening of voice than we do to what is said by the individual. When our body reacts, we feel it and afterward build up our very own story. That is the way we either feel that we can be near individuals, or we feel that we ought to be truly separating. The hidden topic here is, there is no social commitment, except if our neuroception gets the highlights of security.

NOTES

Chapter 2:
The Vagus Nerve

The vagus nerve is known as the longest and most complex of the 12 pairs of cranial nerves, and it originates from the brain. It is in charge of the transmission of information to or from the brain to tissues and organs connected in the body.

It was originally cited as "pneumogastric" before the name "vagus," which came from the Latin term which literally means "wandering," was adopted. This is because the vagus nerve has the longest and most diverse pathway around the body, and it is believed, it "wanders" into tissues and organs in the neck, chest, and abdomen from the brain.

It is the 10th cranial nerve and thus known as the "10th cranial nerve" or "cranial nerve X."

The vagus nerve has sensory nerve cell bodies that come in two bunches, and it serves as a connection between the brainstem (from which it originates) to the body (to which it extends to). It allows the brain to receive information and monitor several of the body's different organic and tissue functions.

The vagus is a mixed nerve that contains parasympathetic fibers carrying somatic and visceral afferents and efferents.

The majority of fibers of the vagus nerve are visceral afferents because of the vast nature of cutting across the thoracic and abdominal cavity, and its internal organs such as the heart, lungs, stomach, gut, etc., and they have a wide distribution that can pass through the central nervous system (CNS). This passage occurs either through the nucleus of the sole tract or monosynaptically. Aside from stimulation of well-defined reflexes, vagus nerve activation produces the manifestation of potentials recorded from the cerebral cortex, the hippocampus, the thalamus, and the cerebellum.

The terminating part of the vagus nerve is called the spinal accessory nucleus.

Etymology

Vagus is a Latin word that means "wandering." It originates from the same root as "vagabond," "vagrant," "divagation," and "vague."

The vagus nerve is most times described in singular terms even though it is paired but sometimes the right and left branches together are called off in the plural as vagi (/ ˈveɪdʒaɪ/ VAY-jy).

The vagus was once historically called the pneumogastric nerve since it was known to be in charge of innervating both the lungs and the stomach.

Structure

Originating from the medulla oblongata, the vagus nerve runs between the pyramid (olive) and the inferior cerebellar peduncle; it extends through the jugular foramen, then passes into the carotid sheath, which is between the internal carotid artery and the internal jugular vein down to the neck, thorax, and abdomen, where it makes contributions to the innervation of the viscera, extending all the way to the colon. That is the reason why it is the longest and most complex of all 12 cranial nerves.

Aside from giving some output to various organs as efferent functions, the vagus nerve is made up of between 80% to 90% of afferent nerves, mostly transmitting sensory information about the state and wellbeing of the body's organs to the central nervous system (CNS).

The vagus nerve comes in a pair; the right and the left vagus nerves, and they descend from the cranial vault passing through the jugular foramina into the carotid sheath, which is between the internal and external carotid arteries, then extends posterolaterally to the common carotid artery. The cell bodies of the vagal visceral afferent fibers are found bilaterally in the inferior vagus nerve ganglia (nodose ganglia).

The right vagus nerve ascends into the neck between the trachea and esophagus when it gives rise to the right recurrent laryngeal nerve and hooking around the right subclavian artery. The right vagus then passes through the anterior to the right subclavian artery, running through the posterior to the superior vena cava, descends posterior to the right main bronchus, and contributes to the complexity of the cardiac, pulmonary, and esophageal plexuses. Forming the posterior vagal trunk at the lower part of the esophagus and it enters the diaphragm through the esophageal hiatus.

The left vagus nerve goes into the thorax between the left common carotid artery and left subclavian artery and descends on the aortic arch, which gives rise to the left recurrent laryngeal nerve, hooking around the aortic arch to the left of the ligamentum arteriosum, which then travels upwards in between the esophagus and trachea. Some thoracic-cardiac branches then branch from the left vagus and further break up into the pulmonary plexus, continuing into the esophageal plexus, and then make an entrance into the abdomen as the anterior part of the vagal trunk in the esophageal hiatus of the diaphragm.

The branches include; Pharyngeal nerve, Superior laryngeal nerve, Inferior cervical cardiac branch, Recurrent laryngeal nerve, Thoracic-cardiac branches, Branches to the pulmonary plexus, Branches to the esophageal plexus, Anterior vagal trunk, Posterior vagal trunk, Hering-Breuer reflex in alveoli

The vagus nerves run parallel between the common carotid artery and the internal jugular vein inside the carotid sheath.

Note; Plexus is a network of an interwoven mass of nerves, blood vessels, or lymphatic vessels.

Nuclei

The vagus nerve includes structurally long, thin fibers called "axons," which originate from the following four nuclei of the medulla:

1. The dorsal nucleus of the vagus nerve – this sends parasympathetic information to the internal organs that lay across the thoracic and abdominal cavity of the body, especially the gut.

2. The nucleus ambiguous – This gives rise to the brachial efferent motor fibers of the vagus nerve and preganglionic parasympathetic neurons that innervate the heart.

3. The solitary nucleus – which receives afferent taste information and primary afferents from visceral organs.

4. The spinal trigeminal nucleus – which receives sensory information about deep/crude touch, pain, and temperature of the

outer ear, the dura of the posterior cranial fossa, and the mucosa of the larynx.

Development

The motor functional part of the vagus nerve is gotten from the basal plate of the embryonic medulla oblongata, while the sensory functional part of the vagus nerve is derived from the cranial neural crest.

Functions of the Vagus Nerve

The vagus nerve is a very diverse nerve, and these are some of its functions:

1. It serves as a tool for the communication between the guts and the brain: The vagus nerve stands as a messenger between the gut and the brain. It conveys information from the gut about how the body is feeling to the brain for processing via electric impulses known as "action potentials."

2. It helps in reducing heart rate and blood pressure: The vagus nerve helps in lowering the heart rate due to its connection to the heart.

The vagus nerve has a close relationship with the heart. It is in charge of controlling the heart rate via electrical impulses to specialized cardiac muscle tissue known as the heart's natural pacemaker, which is in the right atrium, where "acetylcholine" is released to slow down the pulse.

3. It helps in fear management: The vagus nerve sends to the brain information from the gut, linked to stress, anxiety, and fear management. This helps a person recover from a scary or stressful

situation when faced or triggered by helping the person maintain calmness.

Best explained by saying that the vagus nerve initiates your body to relax.

When the sympathetic nervous system pours the stress hormone, cortisol, and adrenaline into your body, in the "fight or flight" responses. It is the vagus nerve that releases acetylcholine into the body, telling the body to relax. The tendrils of the vagus nerves extend to many organs and act like fiber-optic cables that send instructions to release enzymes and proteins like prolactin, vasopressin, and oxytocin, which calm you down. Vagus nerve response varies from individual to individual; for example, people with a weaker vagus response find it difficult to recover from injury, stress, or illness, while people with a much stronger vagus response may find it less difficult to recover rapidly.

4. Balancing of the nervous system: The nervous system is made up of two areas; first, the sympathetic area, which is responsible for the increment of alertness, energy, blood pressure, heart rate, and breathing and second, the parasympathetic in which the vagus nerve is heavily involved in, which helps in the decrement of the heart rate blood pressure, and alertness and it also helps with calmness, relaxation, and digestion. Therefore, the vagus nerve aids defecation, urination, and sexual arousals. Thereby helping to maintain a balance in the nervous system.

Mind you, even though it helps maintain balance in the nervous system, overstimulation of the vagus nerve can cause loss of consciousness

5. It helps in strengthening memory retainment: When the vagus nerve is stimulated, it releases into the amygdala the neurotransmitter norepinephrine, which helps strengthen memories. This, according to research and study, suggests a promising future treatment of conditions like Alzheimer's disease.

6. The vagus nerve prevents and decreases inflammation: The vagus nerve sends anti-inflammatory signals to other parts of the body. Inflammation is a physical condition that is sustained during or after injury or illness, and it is normal to have a certain amount of it, but too much inflammation is linked to many serious diseases and conditions, ranging from sepsis to the autoimmune condition rheumatoid arthritis. The vagus nerve gets a signal at the slightest detection of inflammation through its operation with a vast network of fibers stationed all around the body's organs.

In detecting the incipient inflammation —the presence of a substance called tumor necrosis factor (TNF)— alerts the brain and sends out anti-inflammatory neurotransmitters that regulate the body's immune response.

7. The vagus nerves help in the breathing process: The neurotransmitter acetylcholine, which the vagus nerve sends as a signal, informs your lungs to breathe, literally. To stimulate your vagus nerve, you can do that by yoga, meditation, abdominal breathing, or holding your breath for four to eight counts.

In summary, the vagus nerve, as described before, is a vast network of nerves that has a pathway to almost all the body's organs. Due to the connection and the active transmission of information from the brain to the organs or from the organs to the brain aids in the other functions as well; gag reflex, satiation after eating, vomiting, and fainting.

Effects of The Vagus Nerve

The vagus nerves have emotional effects on the body as well as physical effects.

1. The overstimulation of the vagus nerve in response to emotional stress can cause the overcompensation of the parasympathetic nervous system function to a strong sympathetic nervous system response linking with stress, which causes "vasovagal syncope." This causes the immediate drop of the blood pressure and heart rate and can cause uneasiness or trembling. During extreme vasovagal syncope, there are restrictions of blood flow to the brain, which leads to a shortage of blood supply to the brain, and one loses consciousness in the process. Although, most times, to make the symptoms subside, one has to sit or lie down for the necessary amount of time. Vasovagal syncope affects young children and women more than men.

2. It can also lead to temporary loss of bladder control under moments of extreme fear. That explains why when a person is faced with extreme situations that cause the person to fear, the person may urinate on himself/herself.

Research has proven that women having had complete spinal cord injury can still have orgasms through the vagus nerve, which can go from the uterus and cervix to the brain.

Vagus Nerve Stimulation (VNS)

The results obtained from the rigorous research and study made on the vagus nerve and its functions have birthed vagus nerve stimulation tested through clinical trials holds promises of a future of treatment and cure of serious, incurable disease.

Vagus Nerve Stimulation (VNS) is a medical procedure whereby the vagus nerve is stimulated either manually or by electrical pulses.

This has been used to try and treat a variety of conditions such as epilepsy, depression, rheumatoid arthritis, etc.

According to research, the effectiveness of Vagus Nerve Stimulation (VNS) has consequently been approved to be used in the treatment of epilepsy and mental illness.

Vagus Nerve Stimulation Implantation

This medical procedure, performed by a neurosurgeon, usually takes about 45-90 minutes with the patient most commonly under general anesthesia. Like with all surgeries, the patient stands a risk of infection, including inflammation or pain at the incision site, damage to nearby nerves, and constriction of nerves.

The medical procedure requires two small incisions for the implantation of the nerves. The first incision is made on the upper left side of the chest where the pulse generator is implanted, while the second one is made on the left side of the lower neck along a crease of the skin, where the thin, flexible wires (known as lead) that links the vague nerve to the pulse generator can be put in.

This device is a piece of metal that is flat and round and measures about 10-13 mm thick and 4 centimeters (an inch and a half) across.

This figure is dependent on the model because new models are much smaller.

The device contains a battery, which is made to last from one to 15 years, and when the battery is low, the device is replaced with a less invasive medical procedure which, this time, requires only the opening chest wall incision.

The device is usually activated after implantation, most commonly two to four weeks after implantation, although in some cases, it may be activated right in the operating room at the time of implantation. The device is usually programmed by the treating neurologist in his or her office with a small hand-held computer, programming wand, and programming software. During the programming, the strength and duration of the electrical impulses are programmed, although the quantity of stimulation varies according to the case but is usually initiated at a low level and gradually increased to a suitable level for the patient. The device works continuously and is programmed to switch on and shut off for specific programmed periods— for example, 25 seconds on and 6 minutes off.

The patients are provided with a Magnet Bracelet (handheld magnet) to control the device at home, in the workplace, or anywhere which must be activated and programmed by the treating neurologist to magnet mode. This works by delivering extra stimulation despise the programmed treatment schedule whenever the magnet is swept over the pulse generator site. To turn the device off, the magnet is held over the pulse generator while the magnet is in position while removing it will continue the stimulation cycle. All these maneuvers performed with the magnet can be done by the patient, family members, friends, or caregivers. Literally, it works like a remote control.

The side effects, most commonly related to stimulation, usually improve over time. These may include any of the following:

Hoarseness in the voice, coughing, tickling of the throat, and shortness of breath are the most common but are usually temporary.

This procedure can be used to treat the following:

1. Epilepsy

Epilepsy is a common condition that affects both ain abnormally and causes frequent unpredicted seizures.

Seizures are unpredictable bursts of electrical activity in the brain that affects how it works temporarily. They are characterized by a wide range of symptoms.

Epilepsy has no definite age at which it can occur, but usually, it starts either in childhood or in people over 60. It's most times lifelong but can get gradually better over time.

The treatment of epilepsy involves a small electrical device that is similar to a pacemaker. Under general anesthesia, the device (which has a thin wire called lead connecting it to the vagus nerve) is placed on the person's chest, which helps to send at regular intervals electrical impulses throughout the day to the brain via the vagus nerve.

Vagus Nerve Stimulation is proven to be effective, although it is faced with side effects:

1. Sore throat

2. Nausea/ Stomach Discomfort

3. Difficulty in swallowing

4. Shortness of breath

5. Change in voice by making it hoarse

6. Slow heart rate.

It is advised to report to your doctor if any of these symptoms start or persist as they may be ways to reduce or stop them.

2. Mental illness

Vagus Nerve Stimulation is used to treat drug-resistant cases of clinical depression, and it is found to help in the treatment in the following:

1. Alzheimer's disease: Since the vagus nerve helps one to make memories. This stimulation of the vagus nerve can release into the amygdala, neurotransmitter norepinephrine which strengthens memories. Thus this holds a promising future of treatment and cure of Alzheimer's disease.

2. Anxiety disorders: The vagus nerve helps in stress, anxiety, and fear management. Therefore, Vagus Nerve Stimulation can help in the treatment of anxiety disorders.

3. Rapid cycling bipolar disorder: This is a pattern of frequent, unique episodes in bipolar disorder. In "rapid cycling," a person with bipolar disorder experiences four or more distinct episodes of mania or depression in one year. It can unpredictably occur at any point and can come and go over many years depending on how well the disorder is being treated; it is not necessarily "permanent." The vagus nerve

has been proven to help in improving one's mood. Therefore, the therapy of stimulating the vagus nerve can help in the treatment of this disorder.

3. Inflammation

Inflammation usually occurs as a reaction to injury or infection. It is a localized physical condition in which part of the body becomes swollen, reddened, and often painful. Since it is known that the vagus nerve helps in decreasing inflammation when the vagus nerve sends an anti-inflammatory signal to the part or parts of the body that needs it. It is believed that Vagus Nerve Stimulation can be used in the treatment of inflammation.

Further research and consideration suggest that since the vagus nerve have pathways to almost all organs of the body, that it holds a promising future in the treatment of the following:

1. Inflammation from Crohn's disease, Parkinson's disease, diabetes mellitus, and rheumatoid arthritis.

2. Intractable hiccups

3. Abnormal heart rhythm and heart failure.

Although we were once saying the same thing for rheumatoid arthritis, now vagus nerve stimulation can be used in the treatment of rheumatoid arthritis, which helps reduce the symptoms to a significant level with no serious adverse side effects. Thus, it is believed that this procedure will be used, in the nearest future, to treat some serious, incurable diseases.

NOTES

Chapter 3:

Polyvagal Theory and Post Traumatic Stress Disorder (PTSD)

I t is clear that unpredictable PTSD has a solid neurological and physiological viewpoint to it. A comprehension of polyvagal theory gives a way to comprehend and enhance the terrible and regularly alarming substantial side effects that people living with complex PTSD endure. With a comprehension of the polyvagal theory set up, it turns into a matter of moral need to apply it to the manifestations and enduring of the individuals who have persevered through ceaseless maltreatment. Frequently during psychotherapy, people may end up encountering flashbacks and re-traumatization and be pitched into the conditions of hyperarousal or separation. This exposition contends that it is morally questionable to put patients through such terrible encounters without giving methods to enhance such terrifying manifestations. Patients are "urged to discuss the most agonizing occasions of their lives without helping them to adjust their excitement. That is clearly retraumatizing. Requesting that individuals remember the most loathsome experiences of their lives without showing them how to have a sense of security and quiet is risky to individuals' wellbeing; it is so off-base" (van der Kolk and Najavits, 2013, p. 521)

Information on the neurophysiological premise of complex PTSD symptomology is the basic way to furnish sufferers with a way to comprehend and adapt to the disrupting indications of injury. An examination into the social commitment framework's job in chemical imbalance (Bal et al., 2010), passionate guideline in marginal character issue (Austin, Riniolo, and Porges, 2007), and dissociative experience (Hart, 2013) recommend that that polyvagal theory can be applied very adequately to numerous clutters and ties numerous appearances of sick mental wellbeing together under a solitary recommended neurophysiological instrument. The polyvagal theory "has given one of a kind bits of knowledge into the job of feeling dysregulation in psychopathology, and into the advancement of unusual examples of autonomic sensory system working in various clinical disorders that before were viewed as disconnected" (Beauchaine, Gatzke-Kopp, and Mead, 2005, p. 181)

Further to its job in psychopathology, the polyvagal theory is a hopeful and positive way to deal with amplifying happiness for the most part in the human populace by applying procedures to down direct the crude, dread, and nervousness prompting old vagal reaction and advance the more current mammalian, social commitment frameworks that energize security and development in ideal social and network settings (Porges W. S., 2015). Information on polyvagal theory can be abused in two different ways: the logical power of the theory concerning the physical symptomology of complex PTSD in this way normalizing it and giving away to change psychological reaction to improve things and also, by taking care of mediations that diminishing the force of disagreeable physical side effects and advance a feeling of control by means of enactment of the characteristic quieting impact accessible from the parasympathetic sensory system.

NOTES

Chapter 4:
Trauma Recovery

Most people who have suffered significant emotional trauma (e.g., the newly bereaved, citizens in war-torn countries, those who have been abused or sexually molested) or physical injury (e.g., extreme abuse, crippling disability) are emerging from their misfortune totally or almost fully. Some, though, do not do as well and, for an extended period, manage to relive the same horrific experiences of debilitating terror, depression, and panic. Their bad experiences have traumatized these latter groups of people.

In the book "Waking the Tiger: Healing Trauma," Levine and Frederick (1997) said it was the result of bottled-up somatosensory symptoms following trauma. "During a traumatic experience, there are three main ways people respond," Levine and Frederick (1997) said. They can fight (confront the situation), flee (get away from the situation), or freeze (be completely overwhelmed to the point of immobility by the predicament). Victims applying fighting or fleeing solutions to a traumatic experience are better at dealing with trauma than people freezing in response to shock (Levine & Frederick, 1997). This condition of suspended animation and paralysis occurs involuntarily and unconsciously. The patient has no means to go through all the usual responses correlated to traumatic events during this frozen condition (Levine & Frederick, 1997). The trapped emotions wreak havoc on the traumatized individual because the victim does not adequately release them. Therefore, the trauma solution is to guide the victim along a path (Experiential Sensation-FELT SENSE) that allows them to perceive and release those emotions that are trapped (Levine & Frederick, 1997). The therapeutic method is acquired from researching how pets rebound from traumatic experiences (Levine & Frederick 1997). Confronting trauma, Levine and Frederick (1997) said, should be mostly at an emotional, limbic level of the brain, not just at a rational, executive level of the brain.

The polyvagal theory, which suggests that trauma has a somatic experiential component, also supports Levine and Frederick's trauma theory in some ways. When, as the polyvagal hypothesis and the theory of Levine and Frederick (1997) suggest, trauma has strong emotional origins, features of partnership frameworks such as the DIR system can be implemented to resolve trauma. After determining the functional, emotional development capacity level of the victim, a DIR practitioner may begin to appeal, build and reinforce discovered areas of weaknesses, allowing the victim to escape from the shackling phenomena of a past traumatic event. Calming the traumatized individual is a tool for regulating traumatized individuals in the DIR toolbox. A calm mind creates an opportunity for further emotional regulation and understanding of deep-rooted feelings, all of which are needed for trauma victims to get out of the shackles of the past and begin to achieve new functional capacity heights.

Other relevant trauma theories include the NARM model, which, focused on the mind, suggests that trauma is associated with maladaptation in the history of the victim's attachment. The PTSD model suggests that trauma victims adopt approaches that have evolved and have been effective in the past for their current problems.

Throughout my view, while attachment and trauma seem like opposite ends of the same psychological spectrum, it is clear that while attachment is mostly optimistic, except in severe attachment/ dependence situations, trauma is almost always destructive, at least until the person recovers. Trauma treatment requires a dedicated practitioner willing to learn from their victims and understand their challenges to develop a suitable management strategy.

Recognizing the signs and symptoms of injury, allowing prompt appointments to a trauma therapist, and incorporating several of the modalities mentioned above will likely yield the best outcome for treating distressed children and adults.

Why is the polyvagal theory very important?

For therapists and pop-psychology enthusiasts alike, understanding polyvagal theory can help with:

- Understanding trauma and PTSD
- Understanding Attack and withdrawal in relationships
- Understanding how extreme stress leads to dissociation or shutdown
- Understanding how to read body language

The truth is that emotions are responses (internal or external) to a stimulus. We sometimes happen out of our awareness, particularly if we are out of contact with our internal emotional life or incongruent with it.

To our bodies, our dominant desire to remain alive is more important than even our ability to think about staying alive. This is where the theory of polyvagism comes into play.

The nervous system always runs in the background, controlling our body functions to allow us to think about other things — like what ice cream we'd like to order or how to get that A in medical school. The entire nervous system works in tandem with the brain and, even if we don't want it, can take over our emotional experience.

A story about a gazelle

Animals are a great example of how we deal with stress because they react primarily without consciousness. They're doing what we'd do if we weren't tamed so well.

You've seen a lioness chase a gazelle if you've ever watched a National Geographic Africa special. A group of gazelles grazes, and suddenly one looks up, hyper-conscious of what's happening around him. The entire group is listening and paying attention.

The lioness ends her pursuit after a moment. She's singled out the gazelle, runs as fast as possible (sympathetic nervous system) until he's caught. He immediately goes stiff (parasympathetic nervous system) when he is captured.

The lioness drags the gazelle back to her cubs, where they start playing with her before heading in for slaughter. If the lioness gets distracted and the gazelle sees a moment of opportunity, he gets up and sprints off again, looking like he came back to life suddenly (back to the sympathetic response of the nervous system).

When the gazelle was captured, his reaction to the shutdown came in with fangs around his neck— he froze. The fight or flight came in when he saw the opportunity to run, so he did.

The polyvagal theory encompasses the three states— connection, difficulty, or run or shutdown.

Here's how it works:

Connection mode or... Rest and relaxation... Or myelinated vagus nerve: Myelinated vagus nerve of the parasympathetic nervous system flowing from the nucleus unclear reaction In non-stressful situations, if we are emotionally healthy, our bodies remain in a state of social involvement or a relaxed, natural, non-freaked-out mood.

I like to call it "connection." By connection, I mean we can interact with another human being "connected." We stroll outside, without doubt, loving our day, dining with friends and family, and feeling natural regarding our body and emotions.

It is also called the ventral vagal reaction, as this is the part of the brain triggered during the process of communication. It's like a normal life green light.

How do you see and feel this?

- We have a healthy immune system.
- We feel normal happiness, open-mindedness, peace, and life curiosity.
- We sleep well and eat normally.
- Our expression is flexible and articulate.

- We have an emotional relationship with others.

- We understand and listen to others more easily.

- We feel calm and rooted in our skin.

Freeze, flight, fight, or puff up... Or the sympathetic response of the nervous system: The sympathetic nervous system is our immediate response to stress, affecting almost every organ in the body.

The sympathetic nervous system causes the state we have all heard of "fight or flight." It gives us the signs to keep us alive.

How is this going to happen? How do you see and feel this?

- To search the atmosphere for real danger, we detect risk and freeze.

- We produce adrenaline, epinephrine, and norepinephrine to help us achieve what we need— get away from our opponent or battle it.

- We're sweating and feeling more mobilized.

- We're feeling anxious, scared, or angry.

- The metabolism slows down as the body is rushed for oxygen.

- Our blood vessels surround the intestines and dilate to the muscles required for running or battle.

- Our muscles may feel rigid, strong, tight, vibrating, doleful, shaking, and heavy.

- Maybe our hands are clammy.

- Our stomach can be knotted painfully.

- Our gestures can be seen as guarding our vital organs with our fists clenched or puffing up to look bigger or stronger.

Some people who have both traumas of attachment and subsequent trauma may experience chronic suicidality and episodes of dissociation that last days to months. Research shows that solutions for the long term include:

Dialectical behavioral treatment

Mentalization-based therapy

Transition oriented counseling where trauma affects the nervous system

If we experience emotional or physical danger, we do the same thing as that gazelle. We alternate between peaceful grazing (parasympathetic mode of connection), fighting or flight (sympathetic system of fighting and flight), or shutdown (parasympathetic mode of shutdown).

The reaction is everything when it comes to trying to understand the situation. Perhaps when they leaped out to scare us, somebody was just playing a game, but we fainted. Whatever the cause, whether or not the accident was malicious, our body switched in shutdown mode; we reported it as an injury. Our body moved to shutdown mode.

Or perhaps the injury incident was life-threatening, and our nervous system reacted to the stimulus accordingly.

No matter what the trigger is, our subconscious concluded that what was going on was life-threatening enough to force our body to run or freeze.

If someone has been through such a traumatic event that their body tips into shutdown mode, any incident that reminds the person of that life-threatening occurrence may again cause them to isolate or break down.

People can even live for days or months at a time in a state of disconnection or shutdown.

At intense, sudden noises like explosions or thunderstorms, vets sometimes feel that. A woman who has been raped may switch to hyper-vigilant or dissociated response quickly if she feels someone is following her. Someone who has been violated may go into shock when even another person begins to yell.

The problem occurs when the initial trauma has not been handled in such a manner as to address the original trauma.

That's what PTSD (post-traumatic stress disorder) is — the overreaction of our body to a small response, either stuck or shut down in combat and flight.

People who experience injury and the reaction to shutdown usually feel guilty for their inability to act while their body has not changed. Often they wish they had fought more in those moments.

Vietnam veterans could believe their comrades who died around them, frozen with terror, lost. Victims of rape may believe that they may have not resisted their attacker because they have frozen.

Victims of abuse can believe that they are not trying to escape from their attacker and are either powerless or failing.

A lot of "pressure" practice, which teaches people to stay in battle and flight mode, aims to keep people out of dissociation in actual life or death situations. Unfortunately, in contrast to elite sports teams or Special Forces, such activities are not popular. The right amount of stress, with good recovery, can lead to higher levels of adaptation of our nervous systems.

Coming out of shutdown mode

So how do we get back out of shutdown mode?

The dorsal vagal system's opposite is the system of social engagement.

So, in short, what fixes shutdown mode is to bring somebody into a healthy social commitment or a proper attachment.

Looking into the nuts and bolts of how this happens in our bodies will help us understand why when the body is in battle, flight, or shut down mode, we feel the way we do physically.

We will learn how to change states as we realize what the body reacts the way it does, like a series of instructions and some basic brain science. We should start moving out of the system of fight or flight, out of the style of withdrawal, and back into the state of social engagement.

Whether we are only developing a bond with a young, nervous client or helping them cope with their most traumatic memories as counselors, it is important to know how to handle the polyvagal systems.

It may also be useful because, in some of these signs, you have just found yourself. Such as, "When I'm with my family, even as an adult when they start fighting, I feel light-headed and detached." If you've experienced some of these issues for yourself, perhaps by counseling and even knowing how it functions, you will get yourself out of a disconnected condition.

Studies show that some parts of the brain, including verbal centers and brain reasoning centers, shut down during the recall of traumatic events (Van Der Kolk, 2006).

That's why it's important to conduct therapy in a safe, healthy way, in a safe, healthy environment, or to come out of shutdown mode. That is why it is imperative to have a positive attachment. Or you run the risk of the person getting retraumatized.

Because I'm a psychiatrist, I'll write this to show how to help a patient switch off shutdown mode.

These tips, however, still apply to those who only understand how the shutdown mode works. And it can even encourage those who feel shut down and continue trying to get back to a balanced style of social engagement.

Have a relationship of trust. Due to the potential of re-traumatization, don't even discuss intensively traumatic events— especially those where you believe disconnect mode has set in until the therapeutic partnership feels deeply linked.

As a psychologist, it's important to allow the client to express things that they couldn't communicate with others— shameful thoughts, rage, sexual response, anything that seems scared to share with others.

Find a quiet center of your own. You're throwing them a lifeline if you can empathize with their distress, stay with them in the moment and help them feel connected during their shutdown. You help them get out of the freeze through social engagement.

Combating the desire to dissociate is essential, no matter how gruesome the topic is. As psychologists, because of the mirror neuron reaction, we might dissociate — to mimic the brain of our client, and because it's easy to imagine it occurring to us when experiencing traumatic pain.

The human experience is so powerful that it rewrites that event in our brain when we re-engage the trauma with someone else to support us, adding to the feeling of being supported in the memory of the trauma. We are creating new neural pathways around the trauma, and we can change the response of our body to it.

Let that guide the client. Don't go looking for a witch. Step into the topic if the client brings it up. But, by asking leading questions and trying to get them to confess, it is harmful to prompt the patient into something that is not there. Do not allow your own experience to lead you to imagine that they have experienced something as well.

Standardize your answers. The whole principle of polyvagism would allow one to say "thank you!" To the organs of us. Even if that process is at times overactive — unwarranted fear or anxiety — which our body watches over us, trying to keep us safe.

The skin is the same as the gazelle, either running away or limping. And in the first instance, gazelles have no concept of what feelings are.

Now that the patient understands that their emotional response has been adaptive, primal, and suitable, we can get rid of the shame caused by their non-reaction.

Support them to understand their frustration. Anger is an incredibly adaptive emotion, and we don't allow ourselves to have it. We think it's bad for anger. Yet rage also tells us where we breached our healthy boundaries.

Anger fills us with the power to conquer the barrier. They would make the person understand that they had to resolve the emotional energy, but at the time they wanted to, the strength could not be reflected.

If we can get a person to recognize their frustration in a meeting, they will see that the traumatic event was not completely unresponsive. If we can help them feel even the tiniest twitch of a micro-expression of anger on their face— the subtle lowering of the internal eyebrows— we will reassure them that in that moment, their body did not completely deceive them.

They should reconcile their desires with their bodies and thoughts. This helps develop a state of congruence— where their inner feelings align specific thoughts to their external displays.

Furthermore, as a dissociative memory is explored, feeling anger and shame reduction allows the memory to change fundamentally.

Introduce the motion of the skin. Since shutdown allows us to stop, it is a great way to reactivate body movements when thinking about the pain and reconnect the body and mind to get them out of shutdown.

One of my clients, for example, was in an incident. When the EMS arrived, she was secured to a gurney for charging into an ambulance's rear. More than the actual accident, she felt pain being stuck on that gurney. She was afraid that she would injure her neck during the whole ride to the hospital, and all the stress about a neck injury led her to be paralyzed in terror.

In the therapy session, even talking about the trauma, her body was stiff, frozen, and dissociated.

I asked her, "During that time, how would you want to move?"She said she wanted to be able to lift her legs. I asked her to move her hands deliberately, attentively, the way she wanted to.

It is necessary to deliberately and gradually do the motion, concentrating on the movement's sensation. That patient felt an enormous energy release. She was able to tell the experience as a story in the subsequent treatments, rather than dissociating.

Making the client push— slow hitting, jumping, spinning, and gradually moving in place— flips the individual from shutdown into battle or flight mode, with the aim being to switch into contact or social engagement mode.

Exercises in body movement can fundamentally change the memory in conjunction with talking to a therapist.

Practice reinforcement. In relationships where one person feels they cannot connect well with the other person, an emotional breakdown can occur.

This behavior was defined as stonewalling by one psychologist, John Gottman. Practicing assertiveness may make the client feel more in control of their psychological situation and feel safe to move into habits of healthy relationships.

Breathing practice, mindfulness, and meditation all play a role in becoming more integrated with your body here and now.

Practice strength training and become a Judo Master. It can be important and educate yourself on how to protect yourself better in the future and also, over time, reset the anxiety cycle.

NOTES

Chapter 5:

The Healing Power of Vagal Tone

T he Polyvagal Theory has effectively linked the physical and emotional. Physical actions can regulate emotional conditions, emotional activities can cause physical responses. For example, deep, forceful, diaphragmatic breathing can initiate a state of deep calm, while emotional reactions can lead to stress, triggering elevated heart rate and respiratory rates and a range of other visceral organ reactions, such as stopping digestion as a form of energy conservation. Given the role of the vagus nerve in mediating both physical and emotional reactions, it is no surprise that the vagus nerve can be engaged to better manage our emotional sense of wellbeing and help alleviate physical problems.

As we have seen, under normal conditions, the calming parasympathetic nervous system is dominant, keeping the body in a state of homeostasis. In this context, a vagal tone is an assessment of the body's readiness to perform certain key functions effectively. An ideal vagal tone maintains a baseline from inputs via the vagus nerve received from the parasympathetic nervous system. Among the most important vagal tone functions is controlling heart rate to keep it from beating too quickly. Vagal activity is key to controlling breathing rate, managing the rate of peristaltic contractions during digestion, and further affecting the sensitivities and inflammation of the digestive tract and functioning of the liver. Vagal tone is also a measurement of emotional stability, as emotions form their basis of normalcy when the dorsal vagal and ventral vagal responses are at homeostasis.

But this is not always the case, especially when emotional reactions ignite physiological responses.

Regulating Emotion

The parasympathetic nervous system follows two pathways. The better known, and far more dominant, is the ventral vagal pathway that controls most of the key organ functions. As noted above, it encourages social engagement and interaction to further secure and stabilize the individual. The more recently recognized but older pathway, the dorsal vagal, controls the emergency freeze response, which causes immobility, lightheadedness, speechlessness, fainting, and shock. While the ventral vagal parasympathetic response is mediated by the neocortex, the newly-discovered and most developed part of the brain, the dorsal vagal parasympathetic response is mediated or activated by the most primitive, reptilian part of the brain.

Malfunctioning of either of these vagal pathways can lead to emotional disturbances, but regulating the vagal tone can moderate them. Brain function, specifically emotional responses and reactions, is directly affected by signals carried by the vagus nerve. Studies have shown that behavioral measures of emotional expression, emotional disturbances, self-regulatory skills, and reactivity may be correlated with baseline cardiovascular levels of vagal tone, leading to the conclusion that cardiovascular vagal tone can indicate how well emotions are being regulated and managed. This perspective was not considered traditionally until the Polyvagal Theory opened this enlightened perspective and continues to encourage further experimentation.

The higher the level of vagal tone, the healthier the baseline condition of mind and body. Therefore, given the direct relationship between physical and emotional conditions, it follows that practicing the exercises to improve physical vagal tone will contribute to the improvement of emotional conditions, returning them to more normal baseline levels.

Emotional conditions that may be the consequence of low vagal tone include anxiety, depression, sensations of stress, fatigue not caused by excessive activity, and sleeplessness. Other, more long-lasting emotional conditions may include Post Traumatic Stress Disorder (PTSD) and Attention Deficit Hyperactivity Disorder (ADHD). While many of these emotional disorders may respond to professional counseling and prescribed medication, hard-to-treat cases may respond favorably to vagal toning activities.

Physical actions that can return the body's emotional and physical reactions to normal baseline levels include Yoga stretches and poses, various forms of meditation, oral exercises to stimulate the vagus nerve in proximity to the vocal cords, cold water to the face, auricular massaging of the ears and earlobes and sides of the neck to stimulate the vagus nerve as it passes through the ears and along the carotid arteries. Practicing mindfulness, or being in the moment is a variation on meditation with awareness of every environment stimulus.

The effectiveness of all of these exercises can be enhanced by managed diaphragmatic breathing with deep, deliberate, thoughtful inhales and exhales, which directly stimulate the vagus nerve. The effect is to slightly increase the heart rate on inhales and lower heart rate back to a healthy or homeostatic baseline on exhales.

When the vagal tone is high, physical and emotional states are normal. With low vagal tone, the consequence of not stimulating the vagus nerve can result in a wide range of emotional disorders and, additionally, can contribute to a sense of apathy, loneliness, isolation, and a host of other negative moods. These are all symptoms of the inability to engage socially and participate in social interaction. This may continue a self-perpetuating downward spiral, with the sense of isolation tending to discourage social interaction and with the disconnection from social engagements furthering the feelings of isolation. Low vagal tone can also cause cardiovascular disorders.

Cardiovascular Applications

The relationship between the vagus nerve and the heart has been extensively researched and verified, with further clarification emerging from the Polyvagal Theory.

To set the stage for understanding this relationship, let's begin with the physical side of the relationship.

The vagus nerve travels from the brainstem and connects with the heart muscle or myocardium on the upper right side of the heart, in a cluster of nerves called the sinus node, for short, or sinoatrial node. Here the vagus nerve acts like a natural pacemaker, regulating the heartbeat. During normal conditions, at times of homeostasis, when there is little or no activity or stress, signals arriving from the brain through the vagus nerve slow the heart rate to less than 100 beats per minute. It is subsequently slowed and regulated, sequentially, by the atrioventricular node, the bundle of His, the right and left bundle branches, and finally the Purkinje fibers at the bottom of the myocardium. Every second or so, the heart muscle contracts, blood is forced out of the ventricles toward the lungs from the right ventricle and into the aorta from the left ventricle.

Now, here is where the relationship between the heart and emotional reactions occur, but first, a quick background. The Polyvagal Theory has added clarity to our understanding of how the autonomic nervous system in primates evolved from the more primitive reptile nervous system. Changes evolved to accommodate the more complex primate nervous system, resulting in increasingly elaborate vagal pathways that control or regulate the heart. There was a transition from the exclusive dorsal vagus nucleus among reptiles to a more elaborate structure in mammals, called the nuclear ambiguous.

This included a connection between the heart and the face that enabled social interactions to influence the visceral or bodily functions and possible dysfunctions. In simple terms, this means that social activity and other emotionally regulated activities could play a role in maintaining control over the heart rate, while conversely, cardiovascular events can directly affect emotions.

Charles Darwin, the founder of evolutionary theory, recognized the bi-directional flow between the brain and the heart that is mediated by the vagus nerve. Darwin understood that facial expressions were a physical manifestation of emotions and correctly surmised that neural pathways were connecting the brain with the heart and other organs that would facilitate physiological responses to emotions. Darwin and those of his time were correct in their estimate, despite not yet knowing that the pneumogastric nerve, later renamed the vagus nerve, had its own private network connection between the brain and the heart, apart from the connections of the action-oriented sympathetic nervous system. Capabilities to elevate and reduce heart rate coexist.

A simple but effective determination of vagal tone is a measurement of the heart rate during inhalation when it should increase slightly above baseline, and then measurement of the heart rate during exhalation, when the heart rate should return to baseline. The different rates of the two heart rates can be used to specify the precise vagal tone.

What does this mean to you?

During times of stress, your physical side may be in a state of elevated heart and respiratory rate, and you may be sweating, feeling a need to exert yourself and take action. In those situations when the cause of the sympathetic response is alleviated, and there is no need to run, or fight, or jump, you can cool things down, calm your body with thoughts of calm, peace, reassurance. Repeat to yourself that everything is okay, under control, and it's okay to relax.

NOTES

Chapter 6:

Autoimmune Responses and Inflammation

A relationship has been established between the autonomic nervous system (ANS) and the body's inflammatory response. It has long been understood that the autoimmune system includes inflammation as part of its responses to infection since inflammation helps trigger many aspects of the body's defense, including the release of macrophages or white blood cells and killer T-cells that identify and annihilate invading microorganisms. But often, the autoimmune system can overreact and overwork, continuing inflammation to the point where it can become damaging.

Non-drug treatments to calm the autoimmune responses are being derived from Polyvagal Theory. One approach is rocking, that is, a rocking motion in a chair or on a cushion. This is believed to have a soothing effect overall and a stimulating effect on carotid baroreceptors. Recall that vagal tone can be increased by massaging the vagus nerve on both sides of the neck, where the vagus nerve runs past the carotid arteries. As a result of steady, continuous rocking several times a day for several days, blood pressure levels are lowered as the relaxation functions of the parasympathetic nervous system are engaged.

Another relaxant of the autoimmune response involves contractions of the pelvic floor in a manner similar to contractions of the diaphragm. But while the diaphragm controls the upper body functions of the lungs and respiratory system, the pelvic floor holds the lower body, including the bladder and colon. An exercise to contract and engage the pelvic floor involves sitting on an exercise ball and feeling the pelvic floor begin to relax and settle into the ball, then trying to tighten it, then releasing it, letting it settle again, and repeating the cycle.

Dr. Stephen Porges, the founder of Polyvagal Theory, also advocates standing on a half-exercise ball with a rounded bottom and flat top, with someone else holding your hand to steady and give reassurance. This not only facilitates the therapeutic benefits of the balancing effort but also introduces a social engagement function, which signals the calming parasympathetic nervous system to initiate the socially engaging and relaxing ventral vagal response.

Added to these targeted, specific exercises can be the group of actions that have been used for other situations where the fight or flight sympathetic nervous system has engaged and needs to be turned down, or whenever the dorsal vagal response creates immobility, lightheadedness, and more severe freeze symptoms. These include Yoga poses and stretches, meditation, vigorous cardiovascular exercises, massage of the neck and ears, cold facial therapy, and, importantly, diaphragmatic deep, conscious breathing.

Autoimmune reactions discussed here are moderate and are not at the level of being serious, chronic, or life-threatening. But in cases of more serious autoimmune disorders, there is no substitute for professional medical treatment. The critical first step is the correct diagnosis of the condition and identification of its cause.

Our contemporary ingestion of medications for numerous conditions, both real and imagined, can lead to bodily reactions, notably autoimmune overreactions. This may be exacerbated by taking herbal supplements, which can conflict with medications being taken, or that might initiate autoimmune disorders on their own:

Herbal supplements are lightly regulated by the Food and Drug Administration (FDA), and marketers may not be fully cognizant of potential side effects. Anyone taking prescription medications should check with their physician or pharmacist before mixing their medications with herbs.

NOTES

Chapter 7:

Clinical Applications of Polyvagal Theory

Facial Expressions, Asperger's Spectrum, and Autism

T he Polyvagal Theory addresses the treatment of autistic and other, less extremely affected Asperger's Spectrum children, with the presupposition that these children's social interaction capabilities are physically undamaged and may be awakened with the right type of stimulation. Given that many of these afflicted children are unable to control their social behaviors, or more precisely, unable or unwilling to activate and use their social behavior voluntarily, the Polyvagal Theory holds that there are ways to stimulate the vagus nerve in ways that can encourage the children to manifest the physical dimensions of social engagement.

The Polyvagal model assumes that for many Asperger's children with social communication deficits, including those at the extreme end who are diagnosed with autism, their social engagement systems are intact and are not missing or have irredeemably damaged components of their central nervous systems.

In recalling the earlier discussion of neuroception, this is a concept with the purpose of analyzing and interpreting certain environmental factors and then initiating either defensive reactions or stimulating the onset of the calming reaction. An example is the function of neural circuits that enable a child to smile and respond positively when they recognize someone familiar but to hesitate or flee from an unknown stranger. These reactions are common among all children and can be overcome by simple reassurances.

But in situations involving Autism and less extreme Asperger's Spectrum disorders, the goal is to find ways to arouse or initiate the positive responses to the familiar and suppress the escape or avoidance tendencies that are almost always functioning. The autistic and Asperger's children, according to Polyvagal Theory, are in a permanent state of fear-inducing unfamiliarity and need to be drawn out.

It has been found that autistic and Asperger's children may be engaged socially by the use of encouraging, reassuring facial expressions, altering neuroception. In test situations, it is found that the social inhibition of children with autism may be less of a physical disorder than a purely emotional reaction to stress. If this is correct, it may be theoretically possible to associate their symptoms with either low-level sympathetic defensive responses to stress and fear or possibly due to dorsal vagal freeze immobilization. The combination of facial expressions, especially wide, sincere smiling and eyes wide open, eye contact, and reassuring speaking, can begin to give autistic children a sense that they can trust someone and begin to socially interact with the person. This is consistent with other studies that have demonstrated that social engagement can contribute to the calming, relaxing parasympathetic response.

In contrast, however, new studies are finding that certain brain anomalies can inhibit facial recognition in autistic children and teenagers. In these instances, there is a physical barrier that increases autism symptoms and reduces the potential for facial expression therapy to be effective.

Vagus Nerve Dietary and Nutritional Influences

Among the newer discoveries that involve the vagus nerve, studies are drawing a vagal connection between what we eat and how the brain responds.

New research into obesity control and the role of various types of diets and foods has identified a unique and important role of the vagus nerve in transmitting data from the stomach to the brain. The vagus nerve connects to nerves in the stomach and sends that afferent data to inform the brain of the caloric value, or potential energy, of the stomach's contents. These data, in turn, causes the brain to either suppress appetite-stimulating hormones when calorie counts are high or to increase these hormones when the calorie content is low.

Controlled studies have been conducted among volunteers who agreed to hospital confinement so their exact consumption behavior can be accurately recorded. The usual method of having study participants record their eating experiences in a diary has been found to be highly inaccurate.

The researchers have discovered that the data forwarded to the brain by the vagus nerve can be distorted by over-processed foods and especially by artificial sweeteners. In the case of saccharine-type sugar substitutes, the part of the brain responsible for decision-making, the striatum, is misinformed, interpreting the afferent information to mean there is a specific energy potential available in the gut. When the expected energy is not available, the brain actually becomes confused and encourages more eating, leading to the ingestion of excessive calories.

In an environment of many, often conflicting, dietary recommendations and claims, each purporting to be ideal diets for health and weight control, these new findings strongly discourage diets overly based on over-processed foods and dietary consumption of artificial sweeteners. Natural, unprocessed, whole foods, long the standard of our evolutionary ancestors, remain the more responsible nutritional choice.

NOTES

Chapter 8:
Yoga Therapy and Polyvagal Theory

Y oga therapy is a recently developing, automatic correlative and integrative human service (CIH) practice. It is developing in its professionalization, acknowledgment, and use with a showed responsibility to setting practice principles, instructive and accreditation norms, and elevating exploration to help its viability for different populaces and conditions.

In any case, heterogeneity of training, poor detailing principles, and absence of an extensively acknowledged comprehension of the neurophysiological systems associated with yoga treatment restrain the organizing of testable speculations and clinical applications.

Currently proposed structures of yoga-themed practices center concerning the combination of base up neurophysiological and top-down neurocognitive components. What's more, it has been suggested that phenomenology and first individual moral request can give a focal point through which yoga treatment is seen as a procedure that contributes towards eudaimonic prosperity in the experience of torment, sickness, or incapacity. In this chapter, we expand on these systems and propose a model of yoga treatment that merges with Polyvagal Theory (PVT).

PVT joins the development of the autonomic sensory system to the rise of prosocial practices and states that the neural stages supporting social conduct are engaged with looking after wellbeing, development, and reclamation. This logical model, which associates neurophysiological examples of autonomic guidelines and articulation of enthusiastic and social conduct, is progressively used as a system for understanding human conduct, stress, and disease.

In particular, we portray how PVT can be conceptualized as a neurophysiological partner to the yogic ideal of the gunas or characteristics of nature. Like the neural stages portrayed in PVT, the gunas give the establishment from which conduct, passionate and physical traits rise. We depict how these two distinct yet closely resembling structures - one situated in neurophysiology and the other in an old intelligence convention - feature yoga treatment's advancement of physical, mental, and social prosperity for self-guideline and strength. This parallel between the neural foundation of PVT and the gunas of yoga is instrumental in making a translational structure for yoga treatment to line up with its philosophical establishments. Thusly, yoga treatment can work as a particular practice instead of fitting into an outside model for its usage in inquires about its clinical settings.

Mind-body treatments, including yoga treatment, are proposed to profit wellbeing and prosperity through reconciliation of top-down and base-up forms encouraging bidirectional correspondence between the cerebrum and body. Top-down procedures, for example, the guideline of consideration and setting of expectation, have been shown to diminish mental worry just as hypothalamic-pituitary pivot (HPA) and thoughtful sensory system movement (SNS), and thusly balance insusceptible capacity and irritation. Base-up forms, advanced by breathing procedures and development rehearsals, have been appeared to impact the musculoskeletal, cardiovascular and sensory system work and furthermore influence HPA and SNS movement with frequent changes in resistant capacity and passionate prosperity.

The top-down and base-up forms utilized at the top of the body treatment priorities list may control autonomic, neuroendocrine, enthusiastic, and conduct actuation and bolster a person's reaction to challenges. Self-guideline, a cognizant capacity to keep up the security of the framework by overseeing or modifying reactions to risk or misfortune, may diminish the side effects of differing conditions.

Versatility may give another advantage of mind-body treatments as it incorporates the capacity of a person to "ricochet back" and adjust in light of affliction as well as unpleasant conditions in an opportune manner to such an extent that psychophysiological assets are rationed. High strength is related to faster cardiovascular recuperation following abstract passionate encounters, less seen pressure, more noteworthy recuperation from ailment or injury, and better administration of dementia and incessant agony. Traded off versatility is connected to dysregulation of the autonomic sensory system through proportions of vagal guidelines (respiratory sinus arrhythmia). Yoga is related to both improvements in proportions of mental strength and improved vagal guidelines.

This article investigates the mix of top-down and base-up forms for self-guideline and versatility through Polyvagal Theory and yoga treatment. PVT will be portrayed in connection to contemporary understandings of interoception as the biobehavioral hypothesis of the "preliminary set," which will be characterized later. This will help spread out an incorporated framework to see which mind-body treatments encourage the development of physiological, enthusiastic, and social qualities for the advancement of self-guideline and strength.

We will look at the union of the neural stages, depicted in PVT, with the three Gunas, a fundamental idea of the yogic way of thinking that portrays the characteristics of material nature. Both PVT and yoga give structures to seeing how basic neural stages (PVT) and gunas (yoga) interface the development and availability between physiological, mental, and conduct characteristics. By influencing the neural stage, or guna transcendence, just as one's relationship to the ceaseless moving of these neural stages, or gunas, the individual learns aptitudes for self-guideline and strength. In addition, these structures share qualities that parallel each other where the neural stage mirrors the guna power, and the guna prevalence reflects the neural stage.

PVT, and other rising hypotheses, for example, neurovisceral combination, help explain associations between the frameworks of the body, the cerebrum, and the procedures of the mind offering expanded understanding into complex examples of incorporated top-down and base up forms that are natural to mind-body treatments. PVT portrays three particular neural stages in light of apparent hazard (i.e., wellbeing, peril, and life-risk) in the conditions that work in a phylogenetically decided chain of command, steadily with the Jacksonian guideline of disintegration. PVT acquaints the idea of neuroception with depicting the subliminal recognition of wellbeing or peril in nature through base up forms including vagal afferents, tangible info identified with outside difficulties, and endocrine components that recognize and assess ecological hazard before the cognizant elaboration by higher mind focuses.

The three polyvagal neural stages, as portrayed underneath, are connected to the practices of social correspondence, guarded procedure of activation, and protective immobilization:

1. The ventral vagal complex (VVC) gives the neural structures that intervene in the "social commitment framework." At the point when wellbeing is recognized in the interior and outside condition, the VVC gives a neural stage to help prosocial conduct and social association by connecting the neural guideline of instinctive states supporting homeostasis and reclamation to facial expressivity and the open and expressive areas of correspondence (e.g., prosodic vocalizations and upgraded capacity to tune in to voice). The engine segment of the VVC, which starts in the core ambiguous (NA), manages and organizes the muscles of the face and head with the bronchi and heart. These associations help prepare the individual towards human association and commitment in prosocial connections and give increasingly adaptable and versatile reactions to ecological difficulties, including social communications

2. The SNS is often connected with battle/flight practices. Battle/flight practices require initiation of the SNS and are the underlying and essential guard procedures enlisted by warm-blooded creatures. This safeguard technique requires expanded metabolic yield to help activation practices. Inside PVT, the enlistment of SNS on guard pursues the Jacksonian guideline of disintegration and mirrors the versatile responses of a phylogenetically

75

requested reaction progressively in which the VVC has neglected to alleviate risk. When the SNS circuit is selected, there are monstrous physiological changes remembering an expansion for muscle tone, shunting of blood from the fringe, restraint of gastrointestinal capacity, an enlargement of the bronchi, increments in pulse and respiratory rate, and the arrival of catecholamines.

This assembly of physiological assets makes way for reacting to genuine or accepted peril in the earth and towards the ultimate objectives of security and endurance. When the SNS turns into the predominant neural stage, the VVC impact might be repressed for activating assets for a quick activity. Though prosocial practices and social association are related to the VVC, the SNS is related to practices and feelings, for example, dread or outrage, that helps to prepare the earth for security or wellbeing.

3. The dorsal vagal complex (DVC) emerges from the dorsal core of the vagus (DNX) and gives the essential vagal engine filaments to organs situated beneath the stomach. This circuit is intended to adaptably react to massive peril or dread and is the crudest (i.e., developmentally most established) reaction to stretch. Initiation of the DVC in resistance brings about an uninvolved reaction portrayed by diminished muscle tone and an emotional decrease of heart yield to save metabolic assets and modification in gut and bladder work by means of reflexive poop and pee to lessen metabolic requests required by processing.

PVT states that through these neural stages: specific physiological states, mental traits, and social procedures are associated, develop, and are made open to the person. The physiological state built up by these neural stages in light of risk or security (as decided through the coordinated procedures of neuroception) takes into consideration or limits the scope of passionate and social attributes that are open to the person

A center part of PVT is that examples of physiological state, feeling, and conduct are specific to each neural stage (for a point-by-point audit of the neurophysiological, neuroanatomical, and developmental natural bases of PVT. For instance, the neural foundation of the VVC is proposed to associate instinctive homeostasis with passionate qualities and prosocial practices that are contradictory to the neurophysiological states, enthusiastic attributes, or social practices that show in the neural foundation of protective procedures found in SNS or DVC initiation. When the VVC is predominant, the vagal brake is executed, and prosocial practices and enthusiastic states, for example, association and love, can possibly develop.

When the SNS is the essential guarded system, the NA kills the inhibitory activity of the ventral vagal pathway to the heart to empower thoughtful enactment, and in turn, social and passionate procedures of assembly are bolstered. On the off chance, the DVC idleness reaction is the cautious system, the dorsal engine core is initiated as a defensive component from agony or potential demise, which means dynamic reaction methodologies are not accessible.

It is imperative to note that the VVC has different qualities that empower mixed states with the SNS (e.g., play) or with the DVC (e.g., closeness). Be that as it may, in these instances of mixed states, the VVC remains effectively available and practically contains the subordinate circuits. When the VVC is pulled back, it advances the availability of the SNS as a guard battle/flight framework. Also, the SNS practically restrains access to the DVC immobilization shutdown reaction. In this way, the significant shutdown response that may prompt demise becomes neurophysiologically available just when the SNS is reflexively repressed.

Vagal Activity, Interception, Regulation, and Resilience

Vagal movement, via ventral vagal pathways, is recommended to be an intelligent guideline for the versatility of the framework where high heart vagal tone is associated with increasingly versatile top-down and base-up procedures; for example, consideration guidelines, full of feeling preparation and adaptability of physiological frameworks to adjust and react to the earth. Vagal control has additionally been shown to relate with differential actuation in mind locales that manage reactions to risk evaluation, interoception, feeling guidelines, and the advancement of more noteworthy adaptability in light of challenge. On the other hand, the low vagal guideline has been related with maladaptive base up and top-down handling bringing about poor self-guideline, less social adaptability, discouragement, conclusive uneasiness issues, and antagonistic wellbeing results remembering expanded mortality for conditions, for example, lupus, rheumatoid joint pain, and injury.

Self-guideline is proposed to be subject to the precision with which we decipher and react to interoceptive data, with more prominent exactness prompting upgraded versatility and self-guideline. Thusly, interoception is viewed as significant in torment, habit, enthusiastic guideline, and solid, versatile practices, including social commitment. Furthermore, interoception has been proposed as key to versatility as the precise preparation of interior substantial states advancing a brisk rebuilding of homeostatic parity.

It has been suggested that mind-body treatments are a successful device for the guideline of vagal capacity, with results encouraging towards of versatile capacities including the alleviation of unfavorable impacts related to social difficulty, the decrease of allostatic load, and the assistance of self-administrative abilities and strength of the ANS crosswise over different patient populaces and conditions.

Polyvagal Theory & Mind-Body Therapies for Regulation & Resilience

Mind-body treatments underscore the development of physical mindfulness, including both interoception and proprioception, joined with the care-based characteristics of non-judgment, non-reactivity, interest, or acknowledgment so as to take part in a procedure of re-evaluation of improvements. While being urged to develop familiarity with BME wonders and boosts, the individual is bolstered in a procedure of re-elucidation or re-direction to such improvements so understanding may happen and flexibility, guideline, and versatility might be cultivated.

This ability to change the relationship and response to BME wonders is believed to be fundamental for self-guideline and prosperity. It has been indicated that patients using mind-body treatments for recuperating revealed both a move as far as they can tell and reaction to negative feelings and sensations similar to the improvement of self-administrative aptitudes in managing torment, enthusiastic guideline and re-examination of life circumstances.

PVT offers knowledge into how to figure out how to perceive and move the hidden neural foundation of any given psychophysiological state may legitimately influence physiology, feeling, and conduct, along these lines helping the individual develop versatile procedures for guideline and flexibility to profit physical, mental, and social wellbeing. As mind-body treatments influence the vagal pathways, they are proposed to shape methods for "working out" these neural stages to encourage self-guideline and strength of physiological capacity, feeling guideline, and prosocial practices.

Ideal neural guideline of the autonomic sensory system and the related endocrine and invulnerable frameworks is encouraged through a dynamic commitment of the VVC by using explicit developments or positions, breathing works on, reciting, or contemplation which influences both top-down and base-up forms.

Versatility is proposed to be cultivated by both downregulating cautious states and supporting greater adaptability and flexibility in relation to different wonders of the BME to advance physiological rebuilding just as positive mental and social states. The individual can figure out how to improve the actuation of the VVC with its homeostatic effect on the living being, similar to increment in the office to move all the way through other neural stages, for example, the SNS or DVC when genuine or seen pressure is experienced.

In total, personality body practices can show the person to make the VVC increasingly open, extend the limit of resilience to other neural stages, change the relationship and reaction to SNS and DVC neural stages that happen as common vacillations of the BME, and how to turn out to be progressively talented at moving all through these neural stages. Breathing moves inside yoga regularly encourage comparable moves in the autonomic state with focalized mental and wellbeing outcomes. These practices may likewise add to our capability to encounter association past social communications or systems and to a progressively all-inclusive and unbounded feeling of unity and association.

NOTES

Chapter 9:

Practical Guide to Applying the Polyvagal Theory

S tanley Rosenberg focuses on the basic intricacies of our lives as individuals and as a society in general. It is not because life is changing more than it has in the past, but the world seems to be going into a stranger form of existence, whereas we try to fix one problem, and it can lead to several unintended outcomes. This makes more grounded people live in anxiety, especially those trying to overcome an overwhelming trauma.

People who work with others going through trauma might need to proceed more slowly, as it is understood that the trauma in a person's body partly exists because the body has refused to let it go.

Stephen Porges developed the polyvagal theory, which looks at the nervous system and exactly how it responds to stress and danger. It is often described as a 3-part hierarchical system, and as the theory describes, the body assesses stress or danger through certain signals from the environment. Basically, if we begin to perceive stress, sooner or later, sympathetic activation comes into play.

The way the brain is wired has not changed much over time. It is designed to protect us from dangers of various forms either by fight or by flight, by activation, or by deactivation. When we encounter danger, the social engagement system is stimulated first; if we find that it doesn't do the trick, our activation system engages. That means we are ready to jump into action, and our heart rate starts increasing. If the threat gets too large to be managed, the body activates the dorsal vagus system as a last resort. This theory can be applied in various situations, as described in the following section.

Anxiety

Anxiety is the body's natural response to stress, and many people experience anxiety from time to time, but that doesn't necessarily mean they have an anxiety disorder. This is because anxiety is basically the feeling of apprehension or even fear of future events. People can become anxious in different places and for different reasons. It could occur because of a job interview or a speech or even the first day of school, either as a student or as a teacher. These make the brain and the mind more fearful and nervous.

It is well known that anxiety and panic attacks have an impact on blood pressure and that the vagus nerve connects to various organs in the body. When an organ is not stimulated by the vagus nerve, it can lead to issues ranging from anxiety to stomach-related problems.

Less stimulated or unstimulated vagus nerve branches could be a leading cause of anxiety and panic attacks.

Let's use this example: if your anxiety's root cause is a stomach issue, then when your vagus nerve is stimulated, your vagal tone increases, helping your stomach and solving your anxiety issue. Now you might be wondering exactly how to increase your vagal tone. There are many activities known to increase vagal tone and activation, and they range from breathing exercises to singing, etc. Although these are fantastic methods for stimulation of the vagus nerve, the best method is through the use of cold therapy/ice.

This is a very practical way of relieving yourself of anxiety using the polyvagal theory. When you expose your vagus nerve to cold conditions, it tends to shut down the body's fight-or-flight response to feelings such as anxiety and panic attacks. For example, placing an ice pack at the back of the neck is sure to boost your parasympathetic nervous system. This calms a person down almost immediately as it reduces the heart rate.

Ice packs aren't the only thing that can be used, as even a cold shower or using ice-cold water on your face accompanied by deep breaths can calm your anxiety.

So next time you feel your anxiety rising or feel a panic attack coming on, go to the freezer and get an ice pack and place it gently at the back of your neck, and don't forget to take deep breaths. In doing so, you'll be able to sense your body calming down.

Depression

The polyvagal theory can be applied to depression in different ways. To understand it better, we have to look at the visceral level of vagal nerve activation through this theory. Mental disorders such as depression are mostly caused by the malfunctioning of the autonomic/vegetative nervous system. Both the parasympathetic and sympathetic systems are dominant, while the vagal tone is low. In depression, there is a constant level of stress which makes a person consistently feel uneasy and prevents them from behaving appropriately.

This is why people suffering from depression lack the passion and drive for many things and are unable to relax. Their sleep is unrefreshing, and they tend to wake up tired. In depression, the "smart vagus" (ventral vagus) system cannot cope with the sympathetic branch of the nervous system.

Naturally, after a stressful experience, the "smart vagus" should be able to enforce a "vagal brake" (vagal stimulation) or sympathetic deactivation, decreasing the heart rate and stabilizing the breathing pattern. However, this action can be blocked by traumatic experiences, and this leads to imbalance. So instead of smart vagus activation, the parasympathetic replaces the sympathetic, and this can lead to apathy in a person.

Breathing exercises are a great way to heal depression for various reasons. The key functions of the autonomic nervous system include regulating heart rhythm as well as breathing. These are both controlled by the vagus nerve. Breathing is relaxed and calm when the smart (ventral) vagus is active, while the sympathetic system handles breathing when under stress by causing shorter and shallower breaths.

When you learn to improve your breathing, you can access the vagal brakes (vagal activation causing sympathetic deactivation). People battling depression would need to change several aspects of their breathing, including taking deeper breaths in order to expand their lung capacity and to increase oxygen metabolism. There are additional benefits to taking deeper breaths, such as building one's self-esteem, confidence, and trust in themselves.

Also, note the quality of the exhale because it also affects the sympathetic system. A relaxed breath doesn't just fill your lungs with oxygen, but it comes with acceptance and trust. Breathing therapy is a good way to let go of all obstacles to focus on achieving relaxed breathing. By doing so, you are letting go of the trauma that causes the failure of the vagal brake. Breathing exercises can help in restoring balance by accessing and healing the vagal brake.

Although this could seem like a stressful way of handling depression, progress is made with each relaxed, deep breath which helps you on your path to recovery in everyday life.

Trauma

People who have unresolved trauma or PTSD from an event in the past may pass through life in a version of constant fight-or-flight. The main challenge with this is that it disrupts your everyday life and affects your daily activities. There are, however, ways to channel this fight-or-flight response into other activities that can be soothing and relaxing.

Activities such as cleaning the house, working out in the gym, going on a run, or gardening, for example, are great channels, but they might feel different if done with the intention of engaging the social engagement system. However, this can be difficult for some trauma victims as their fight-or-flight sensations cannot be channeled effectively. This causes the body to shut down and make them feel trapped.

If you feel depressed, shut down, and dissociative because of trauma, getting in touch with your fight-or-flight response could prove positive. A good way is through body awareness techniques which are a part of cognitive-behavioral therapy (CBT) and dialectical behavior therapy (DBT). These therapies can help you slowly move away from your shutdown or dissociative responses and become more engaged.

Shutdown responses can be eradicated by understanding your body and becoming more present while being able to attend to momentary muscular tension. Mind and body therapies help in a wide range of areas in health and well-being.

These therapies can help reactivate a person out of shutdown and can encourage the shifting to fight-or-flight responses. Both CBT and DBT help teach individuals to assess their safety better. There is a possible link to feeling safe enough and moving into social engagement activation.

Some of the physical symptoms of trauma include tightness in the chest, exhaustion, and a sinking feeling in the stomach, among others. Massage, tai chi, acupuncture, and counseling, for example, are great mind and body therapies that make us feel more in control and calm.

Autism

The polyvagal theory offers a good explanation for most common autistic features such as social difficulties, sensory sensitivity, and gut dysfunction while at the same time proposing strategies to ease the severity of certain features.

Due to the evolution of mammals, parts of the autonomic nervous system came to be integrated with neural pathways that have control over the face and the head. This makes the ANS a great asset to the control and regulation of senses other than the two common ones. This new circuit is very relevant to the polyvagal view on autism as it can inform more primitive circuits and has also evolved to enable prosocial behaviors.

The vagal pathway also involves a new system that originates in a part of the brain stem, and this helps in controlling muscles of the face and head and also handles facial expressions, speaking, listening, and ingestion. It allows for vocalization and facial expressions, which are powerful approaches to engage in different social behaviors.

When this system is shut down, it results in many of the traits present in autism, such as poor vocal intonation, lack of facial expressions, hypersensitivity to sound, gut problems, defensive stares, and selective eating, among others.

Just as humans are social animals and look at trusted people for safety cues, it may be more difficult for autistic people who neither recognize nor respond to these cues. This is why their bodies detect danger in social engagements.

Transcutaneous vagus nerve stimulation is one way of working with autism. This is a technique whereby an electrical current is applied to the vagus nerve. This nerve runs between the brain and different areas of the body like the heart, the skin, and the gastrointestinal tract. As previously mentioned, the vagus nerve is very important to both the physical and emotional responses in the body and enters either fight-or-flight mode or rest-and-digest.

The vagus nerve can be stimulated electrically through an implanted device or an external device applied to the skin. If you think this sounds dangerous, you should know that vagus nerve stimulation is an FDA-approved treatment for seizures, and research has shown that this same treatment can be used for depression.

Different research studies have shown that when treated with thoracic vagus nerve stimulation (TVN), children with autism have shown improvement in their behaviors, cognitive functions, and, of course, seizure frequency.

How to Optimize Your Autonomic Functioning Using the Polyvagal Theory

During the last trimester in utero and the following year after birth, the autonomic nervous system undergoes rapid changes. These changes are necessary so infants can breathe, maintain body temperature, obtain food, and much more. Such development is the basic progression in the biology of infants to regulate their physiological and behavioral state when interactions with another person take place, which is most likely the mother at first.

It is thought that these developmental changes and their neural pathways, which regulate the autonomic state, can provide a neural platform in supporting the abilities of infants to be expanded when they engage with objects as well as people in a frequently changing environment. This causes the emerging behavioral patterns and social interaction needs and desires of a growing infant to be viewed within the context of maturational alterations in their autonomic nervous system.

Since the autonomic nervous system plays a crucial role in a child's survival when they transition from the prenatal to the postnatal environment, it is quite astonishing that the central mechanisms of the autonomic nervous system have been digressive to pediatric medicine.

The nervous system of mammals did not just develop for the sole purpose of surviving in life-threatening and dangerous situations but also to promote social interactions and bonding. To achieve this adaptive flexibility, a new neural strategy seeking safer environments has been developed while the more primitive neural circuits regulating defensive approaches have been retained. To accommodate both fight-or-flight as well as social engagement behaviors, the modern vagal system in mammals has evolved to enable rapid, adaptive shifts in more autonomic situations.

Three Organizing Principles

There are 3 organizing principles when it comes to the polyvagal theory, namely hierarchy, neuroception, and co-regulation.

Hierarchy

The autonomic nervous system responds to sensations in the body and signals from the environment with one of 3 different responses. These pathways are activated in a particular order, the order of evolution when it comes to responding to challenges predictably. They include the dorsal vagal branch, which has to do with immobilization, the sympathetic nervous system for mobilization, and lastly, the ventral vagus branch, which is in charge of social engagement and connection.

Neuroception

This is a word coined by Dr. Porges himself, which he used in describing the various ways the autonomic nervous system responds to people or situations that appear safe, dangerous, or life-threatening situations.

Co-regulation

Co-regulation describes how an individual's responses are influenced by the responses of another person. The polyvagal theory identifies co-regulation as an important biological response as it is viewed as necessary to sustain life. Through this reciprocal regulation of various autonomic states, we decide whether we feel safe enough to want a connection and create and sustain certain relationships. The autonomic nervous system is thought of as a foundation upon which all life experiences are built. It is viewed as the platform upon which we base all our experiences. The various movements we make in the world, such as connecting and isolating, coming and going, etc., are all directed by the ANS.

With supportive, co-regulating relationships, we tend to become much more resilient. These relationships help us master the art of survival, and that is why the ANS is continually learning habits of creating connection and protection in relationships.

It is hopeful to say that early intervention can help shape the nervous system, as can ongoing experiences. As we know, the brain continuously adapts our responses to different environments and experiences. The ANS is very engaged, and we, too, can influence it as we please. Our nervous system is built to reach out for co-regulation as we experience moments of either safety or danger. The signals conveyed, either of safety or of danger, which are sent from one autonomic nervous system to another, can regulate or increase certain reactions.

Optimizing Autonomic Function

Optimizing your autonomic functioning can be done through taking deep breaths, box breathing, cold/ice, and gut health.

Deep Breathing

Although this might seem cliché, there is a connection between respiration and heart rate, which affects the vagus nerve. This is a good reason why yoga can help reduce overall stress. Breathing exercises can increase vagal tone and help in managing blood pressure.

Box Breathing

When having a panic attack, you can try box breathing as follows:

Inhale and count to 4

Hold and count to 4

Exhale and count to 4

Wait and count to 4

You can repeat these steps until you are in control again.

The reason this helps is that the slow expansion of your lungs can send signals to slow down your heart, and this can help calm your entire body, including your nervous system. The vagus nerve connects the signaling and releasing of acetylcholine which is a calming chemical that helps the body relax.

Remember the Cold?

Never forget that cold tunes the vagus response, and this can slow down sympathetic nervous system activation. Cold exposure can help in relieving depression and anxiety. When you stimulate the vagal pathway, you also stimulate digestion. Cold exposure can reactivate the gastric nerves.

Take Care of Your Gut

Did you know that microorganisms in the digestive system communicate with the brain? The microbiome can be said to be the ecosystem of good bacteria present in your body and on your skin. Most times, when people talk about this, they are referring to the microbes in the colon and intestines.

There have been studies on animal models as well as some human evidence that when the microbiome is thriving, it can boost mood and reduce anxiety. To determine if the vagus nerve was the reason for this, experiments were conducted on rodents with and without a vagus nerve. The ones with the vagus nerve seemed to experience reductions in anxiety as well as depression indicators, unlike those without.

Developing Your Child

As a parent, you can help build the autonomic system of your child and tune their vagal pathways through loving care and bonding.

Giving your kids cold showers shouldn't be the first step, as you should wait until they know that's what they want. During the infant stage, baby massages and skin-to-skin contact can help develop the baby's vagal tone. Once children are older, other ways to help tone their vagus nerve are cold blast showers and breathing techniques. Other ways to develop this include yoga, massage, and mind-body techniques. The benefit of toning the vagus nerve is that it extends to the major organs in the body.

Surgically Implanted Electrical Vagus Nerve Stimulator

The vagus nerve can be activated surgically in order to more aggressively treat a dysfunction. There are surgical implants to stimulate the vagus nerve, such as electric stimulators for patients who suffer from severe epilepsy or depression.

Find Your Safety Cues and Train Them

Finding your safety cues and training them with a little practice can help you feel safe. Your safety cues can keep your anxiety and fear responses from kicking in. A good way to go about this is finding your safe place or your happy place when you are calm. To do this, imagine you are in the place you feel most at ease and peaceful. Ensure to make use of sensory information as much as possible such as smells, sounds, and sights, and practice this visualization often. Then when you begin to experience fear or anger, you can initiate your safe place visualization with little effort.

NOTES

Conclusion

T he polyvagal theory has had a global impact on both clients and counselors; many counselors have used this theory to improve many health statuses. Many of the things stated help us in facing the reality of life, including putting a smile on our faces, dancing out stress, singing, playing an instrument, having a correct state of thought, being among positive people, knowing how to control your body to not enter into trauma and reaching out to a counselor. All these are very true to help everyone in any kind of distress. Based on this theory, Porges has been able to break down music therapy into behavioral processes to encourage social engagement into action and to find out how clients react behaviorally and physiologically.

When calm, there is a physiological regulation in our behavior. We have also learned that a mechanical change in our breathing has an increase in the influence of calming and a good health benefit to the vagus nerve. This has helped in reducing the number of health attacks we had back then. Also, try from now on to be positive once finished with this book. Don't ever say, "it will never work" or "I can't." When we change all these thoughts, sooner or later, you will appreciate the theory. Try to always look out for neighbors who have a similar problem to the ones stated and help them out with this exercise; it could also be a practical way to see how the polyvagal theory works. It is also important to keep records as a client on how it has changed your health.

The normal functioning of the body is regulated by what Stephen Porge calls the "Social Engagement System" (social communication). This vagus system enables us to interact and communicate with other people from birth. But when we are stressed, it diminishes our ability to do that.

He/she should take advantage of breathing exercises. Since the vagus is active when the breaths are calm and the sympathetic system is active when the breaths are distorted, short and shallow breaths tend to create a form of imbalance in the nervous system. Depressed people should learn to change their breathing habits by taking longer inhales to stretch the capacity of the lungs to take in more oxygen and longer exhales for relaxation.

For autistic people, while growing up, their body system was immobilized. The consequence is that they became agitated, have difficulties digesting food, and their interactions with the outside community are distorted.

So there is a beautiful ray of hope for autistic patients. Through several therapies and counseling sessions, people suffering from autism can learn to reconnect with their brain and body, gain mastery over it, and above all, feel safe and secure in this beautiful world of ours.

To give you the needed time to digest all the information you've absorbed from this book, I will end my tirade here. I hope this book has taught you all you need to know about the polyvagal theory.

NOTES

The Vagus Nerve

Erika Newton

Introduction

O ur body is a wonderful system, yet, many fail to take care of this system well. We let it slow down and become destroyed from within. We mostly react rather than being proactive about our health. Instead, we need to focus on the vagus nerve.

Most of you might are thinking, just what is this vagus nerve? What purpose does it serve? How is it related to taking care of my body?

We are going to look into great detail about the vagus nerve. But for now, know that this nerve is an important nerve that you probably have not heard of before. Some of its functions include regulating blood glucose and blood pressure, releasing testosterone and bile, promoting healthy functions of the kidneys, and even assisting with saliva secretion. And these are just some of its functions.

This book is your guide to becoming more aware of the vagus nerve, finding out how it can help you, and learning the details about it. There is a lot to cover, so let's begin with what the vagus nerve is and dive into its functions.

Within our bodies, we have different nerves. There are nerves that extend from our brain called cranial nerves, and the vagus nerve is one of these 12 nerves. However, it's more than just that. It's not only one of the 12 cranial nerves, but it's also the longest. The name comes from the Latin vagus nervus, meaning "wandering nerve," since it tends to "wander" from our brain stem all through the organs in the chest cavity, abdomen, and neck.

Now, what's in this area? Our heart, lungs, and digestive tract are all parts of our abdominal cavity and chest cavity. The vagus nerve takes care of the vital functions of these different areas of the body.

It has a big responsibility. It isn't just a huge nerve; it's a nerve with a whole lot of responsibility.

The vagus nerve is responsible for your digestive, immune, respiratory, and cardiac systems. However, there's so much more to it. It's vital a long nerve that helps the brain communicate with everything in the body, whether it be breathing, heart rate, or other bodily functions.

There is a lot to this nerve; for the most part, it is responsible for the parasympathetic functions of the nervous system.

But what exactly does that entail? Read on to find out.

Chapter 1:
What is the Vagus Nerve?

Y our whole body, from head to toe, is full of nerves. These are effectively the main reason you control your body and how your body interacts with other items as well: your body interacts with a stimulus, and your nerves report that stimulation back to the brain for processing. Your nerves are also directly responsible for making sure you can control your body; when you want to act on something, your brain processes the request and sends it to the brain via the nerves.

The vagus nerve is just one of those nerves. It begins at the brain and drops down through the body, allowing for the quick transmission of stimuli from the body to the brain and from the brain to the body. We will take quick look at how nerves function and why they are critical. We will address the cranial nerves, thirteen pairs of particularly important nerves. Finally, we will see what happens when the vagus nerve is not functioning.

Nerves

Nerves are highly specialized cells designed to send impulses. These impulses send information from one nerve to the other to get the message to where it needs to go. These impulses called action potentials are effectively the activation of a nerve via chemicals that then sends an electrical impulse down the nerve to pass it along.

These impulses travel from nerve to nerve, much like a student in a classroom passes a message to their neighbor to get the note sent to the right person on the other side of the room. Your brain, however, is passing these notes on an entirely different level. To present you an idea of just how much is going on in your brain at any given time, imagine the following:

You have 100 billion neurons

Each fires up to 200 times per second

Each impulse travels to 1000 other neurons

So, to see just how many impulses occur, you must multiply 100,000,000,000 by 200 by 100, and the answer is 20,000,000,000,000,000. That is an incredibly intimidating number—it is 20 million billion. Your brain is moving around up to 20 million billion impulses of information within a second.

Your nerves are meant to take these impulses from a place nearly instantaneously—and they get quite close. What starts out as an electrical impulse on the end of an axon creates a release of chemicals that interacts with the other nerves in line; and this happens over and over, spreading to upwards of 1000 neurons per firing. This means that the transmission of information flies across the brain incredibly quickly.

The Cranial Nerves

Nerves come in two forms—spinal nerves and the cranial nerves. The only difference is the source of origination. The spinal nerves go from the spine to various parts of the body. The cranial nerves, as you may imagine, go from the brain directly to various portions of your upper body. Primarily, these go to the head, your neck, and torso. Each cranial nerve comes in a pair and serves a different function.

Cranial nerves are usually either responsible for sensing, such as transmitting information about what your body is interacting with, or for motor purposes, or controlling a function. This means that each nerve will have its own primary specialty and will perform differently. When you are reading or learning about cranial nerves, you may see them referred to as Roman numerals from I to XII to denote their locations. I is the closest to the front of the head in origin while XII will be the furthest from the head. Ultimately, the vagus nerve is designated as X.

The Sympathetic and Parasympathetic Nervous Systems

Your body has two primary modes. In the fight or flight mode, your body is incredibly active and ready to fight. There is the rest and digest mode, in which your body is able to slow down and properly process food. These are both a part of the autonomic nervous system—the part of the nervous system primarily ruled by the peripheral nervous system or the part outside of the brain. The autonomic nervous system, in particular, is responsible for the unconscious portion of the body. Effectively, it is those parts not controlled by you but are critical for being kept alive.

Your body's functions are primarily divided into conscious movements and unconscious movements. Your conscious movements are actions you personally choose to do; they are primarily voluntary and not critical to living such as choosing to walk around or actively deciding to go somewhere or jump. They can only happen when you are conscious.

Your unconscious actions, on the other hand, must continue even when you are asleep or unconscious. These are regulated behaviors, such as the heart beating and the body digesting its food. If you had to be conscious to breathe and control your heart, you would literally never be able to sleep without dying.

The sympathetic and parasympathetic nervous systems are a part of this unconscious system. Your parasympathetic nervous system keeps you calm, activating the rest and digest mode. When your vagus nerve is activated, you automatically begin to self-regulate. Your parasympathetic effectively suppresses the sympathetic nervous system, creating a calming effect. It is absolutely critical because your body cannot effectively digest while also actively attempting to flee or fight off a threat. During this stage, as you relax, more blood is diverted to your guts to help regulate and slow down the functions of the body that control healing, resting, and processing food.

The sympathetic nervous system is the one that reacts when you are exposed to a threat. When you feel a threat to yourself, your body immediately activates the sympathetic nervous system in preparation. With the sympathetic nervous system activates, your body is prepared to tackle anything thrown your way. In short, you are ready to fight or run. Blood is cycled through your body quicker as you breathe more, enabling your body to have the oxygen necessary to respond quickly and stay on your feet. Effectively, the sympathetic nervous system prepares your body for vigorous activity.

The Vagus Nerve and Bodily Regulation

The vagus nerve itself is surprisingly diverse. While most of the cranial nerves are designated for either sensory or motor functions, the vagus nerve is responsible for both. It is known as sensorimotor. The vagus nerve receives and sends all sorts of information. Of all of the cranial nerves, the vagus nerve is the longest—it goes from the medulla, a portion of your brainstem, all the way down through your neck and torso, and to your abdomen.

The vagus nerve has four distinct purposes as it brings information back and forth. They are critical in regulating the body. In particular, the vagus nerve is responsible for:

- Sensory input: the vagus nerve transmits feedback from the heart, lungs, throat, and abdomen to the brain to help the brain know how best to regulate

- Taste input: the vagus nerve helps with the sensation of taste

- Motor function: the vagus nerve is responsible for controlling the muscles in the throat needed for both swallowing and speaking

- Regulating the parasympathetic nervous system: the vagus nerve is responsible for regulating digestion, breathing, and heart rate

These four purposes can be broken down into several functions. In total; there are six within the categories of the four functions:

- Triggering anti-inflammatory reactions: the vagus nerve is responsible for telling the body when to stop inflammation by sending out anti-inflammatory messages for the rest of the body.

- Regulation of the sympathetic and parasympathetic nervous systems: these systems are designed to control how alert or relaxed the individual is. They control whether you are in fight or flight mode or if you are in rest-and-digest mode. If your sympathetic nervous system is active, your body is in fight-flight-freeze mode, and when your parasympathetic nervous system is in control, you are calmer and more relaxed.

- Brain-gut communication: the vagus nerve allows for communication from the gut to the brain.

- Regulating circulatory system: our heart rate and blood pressure are directly related to your vagus nerve. The activation of the vagus nerve slows down the heart rate.

- Managing anxiety: when you are anxious, it is usually because the vagus nerve is not able to regulate itself properly, and in response, the individual feels anxious even when they do not need to.

- Allowing for relaxation: because the vagus nerve activates both the sympathetic and parasympathetic nervous systems, it allows for relaxation in certain scenarios. If you need to relax, you activate the parasympathetic nervous system.

The Vagus Nerve and Mind-Body Communication

Because the mind and body are so incredibly intertwined, they need some way to directly communicate. This is the main reason why the vagus nerve is so important: it allows for communication between the mind and the body. The nerve receives signals from the body, and then translates them for the mind to receive. The vagus nerve, in particular, is designed to facilitate that communication. It provides all the feedback for the brain to determine whether the body is functioning properly or if the instructions to the body need to be changed in any way.

Effectively, the nerve acts so that the mind can directly interact with the body and regulate it, allowing always to function properly. This means that the vagus nerve, with its connections to the lungs, the heart, and the digestive tract, is responsible for ensuring that your brain keeps your body alive. Without this nerve, your brain would not know how to regulate itself.

The Vagus Nerve and Emotional Control

Beyond being responsible for your physical bod, the vagus nerve is also critical when it comes to emotional self-regulation. Because the vagus nerve interacts with your sympathetic and parasympathetic nervous systems, it is closely related to whether you are feeling relaxed or anxious. In particular, the stimulation of the vagus nerve seems to have a calming effect on the entire body. When you stimulate the vagus nerve, you are able to directly relax. You are triggering all of the chemicals of the body that slow the heart rate and therefore calm the body.

Think about how people say that yoga is incredibly calming or they rely on techniques such as deep breathing as it helps them feel more stable and in control. This is because it triggers the vagus nerve which in turn triggers the heart to slow down. As such, the body calms down. There is no reason for alarm or feeling anxious. Effectively, the vagus nerve is like a magic switch that enables you to suddenly calm down to get through those difficult emotions that could otherwise become problematic.

Your whole body, from head to toe, is full of nerves.

Chapter 2:
Important Functions of the Vagus Nerve

O ur body functions optimally like a symphony orchestra. Each of the various instruments has specific parts to play, and optimal harmony can only be achieved if each instrument is directed toward doing its job. The orchestra's conductor ensures that no instrument is off-tune or tempo, as a single error could lead to a terrible performance. A conductor that does not keep its goal will also result in a broken performance.

The vagus nerve is the conductor of a symphony orchestra for the human body. It controls the activity of so many different organs and cells, but only when it functions optimally. The body's multiple organs and cells must be capable of detecting and communicating different signals correctly. Dysfunctional signaling can result in a loss of equilibrium in the system, and ultimately a disorder and disease.

The vagus nerve (vagus, from Latin, wanderer) is called that because it is connected to almost all the organs in the body, not just one; it is everywhere. It is responsible for sending sensory information to the central nervous system. It may be considered as the wire conducting electricity from the organs to the brain and vice versa. If that wire breaks somewhere, the organ function will be compromised or lost. For instance, your wounds may not heal fast, you cannot sleep, you eat too much or too little, you feel over-anxious, and the list goes on forever.

Let's break down all of the various functions the human body that orchestra conductor performs for the vagus nerve.

Sensations of the Ear

This branch's function is pure sensation, allowing us to feel pressure, touch, temperature, and moisture on each of the ear's central segments. This is clinically relevant and quite significant, as this is one of the major areas where the VN can be activated, using therapies such as acupuncture.

Allowing Food to be Swallowed

The second function of the VN (the pharyngeal branch) regulates the activation of five pharynx muscles: the three constrictor muscles at the back of the throat and two other muscles that link the throat and the soft palate (the soft tissue at the back of the mouth's roof). These muscles are involved in the pharyngeal process of swallowing, which includes moving chewed food towards the larynx and the esophagus while holding it out of the trachea, thereby keeping the airways free. The active motor part of the gag reflex is also regulated by this VN branch.

Managing Your Airway and Vocal Cords

Are you conscious of the effort required to keep your upper airways open with every breath you take? The muscles involved in this process are also involved in voice development. If you have ever wondered what nerve is responsible for ensuring verbal communication with those around you is feasible, it's the vagus!

The superior and frequent laryngeal nerves are the third and fourth branches of the VN. The muscles above the vocal cords are responsible for the superior laryngeal branch, while the recurring laryngeal branch is responsible for the muscles below the cords.

The superior branch of the laryngeal carries motor information to the larynx muscles to control vocal pitch. The suboptimal feature of the superior branch of the laryngeal results in a pitch transition. A chronically hoarse voice or an easily fatigued, monotonous voice is a sign of poor vagal tone (signaling capacity). Irritation of this nerve can also lead to a cough and the risk of aspiration (i.e., food or drink entering the trachea by impaired vocal cord function).

The recurrent laryngeal branch carries motor information to the muscles below the vocal cords, allowing the vocal cord structures to form sounds by opening, closing and tensioning. It also has a sensory component that relays information from the esophagus, trachea, and internal mucous membranes. Any dysfunction of these nerves during physical activity contributes to heaviness, speech loss and trouble breathing.

Controlling Breathing

What about taking a breath? Okay, the vagus also has a role to play in managing this vital function. The VN's pulmonary branch runs into the pulmonary plexus, connects to the sympathetic nervous system, and innervates both lungs' trachea and bronchi. The vagus component is a sensory nerve that relays information about lung expansion levels to the brain, as well as the levels of oxygen and carbon dioxide.

Vagus tone is expected in the pharynx, larynx, and trachea to open the airway. The pharynx and larynx muscles are innervated by the VN motor components. The suboptimal activity of these neurons can lead to obstruction of the airways, as occurs in chronic obstructive pulmonary disease (COPD) and obstructive sleep apnea. Both symptoms are a sign of low vagal tone and activation of the vagus nerve.

Controlling Heart Rate

Your heart beats to fill oxygen into your tissues and to take toxins away to the organs that dispose of them. The VN plays an important role in ensuring the heart rate stays within a comfortable range when the body is not under threat. Without the VN, the heart would not be working close to its optimum pace.

The sympathetic nervous system activates the heart during fight-or-flight times to increase its pumping rate and the pressure of the contractions in both ventricles. After the stressor passes, the rest-and-digest phase takes over, and the body moves towards the phase of vagal activation. At this time, the VN's parasympathetic fibers slow the heart rate and actively lower the pumping contraction pressure. These fibers work to lower heart activity, allowing the heart to rest and recover from stressful times and severe activation.

Maintaining Optimal Blood Pressure

Blood pressure is an important determinant of the amount of fluid in the bloodstream. The kidneys function to filter the body's fluid and toxins and thus are the major manager of the blood pressure in the body. The vagus nerve relays information from and to the kidneys to help it control the flow of water and urine from within the kidney glomeruli, the kidney's essential filtration unit, while it controls the body's internal blood pressure. When the body is under stress, the vagus and sympathetic nerves draw signals from the blood vessels (in particular the carotid body) and relay them up the brainstem and back down to the kidneys. The kidneys then restrict their blood vessels and increase blood pressure by reducing the amount of water being filtered out through the bloodstream. When the body is calm, carotid body impulses instruct the kidneys to pump out more water to relieve blood pressure.

High blood pressure is a normal condition, and medications are often used to regulate it. It can be a symptom of the overactivation of the stress hormones of the adrenal glands and the stress response of the sympathetic nerves. It is also a very common sign of damaged vagus nerve and poor vagal tone.

Managing Hunger and Satiety

Satiety is attained when the brain receives vagus nerve signals. We require signals from the liver to be satiated, indicating we have enough fat, protein, and carbohydrates in the body. Both carbohydrates and fats are metabolized in the liver.

The following control is mediated by the vagus nerve for carbohydrate metabolism: when blood sugar levels gradually decrease, afferent vagal fibers in the liver increase activity and signal to the brain that more carbohydrates are required by the liver cells. Nevertheless, this mechanism does not signal abrupt changes in blood sugar; these are detected immediately within the brain.

The small intestine releases a hormone called glucagon-like peptide 1 (GLP-1) as a response to increased levels of blood sugar which the body translates as satiety. Diminishing levels of GLP-1 signal the vagus nerve, which in turn manages a slow reduction of blood sugar. Many pharmaceutical companies are now producing medicines that work along the GLP-1 pathway to help manage hunger; however, activating the vagus nerve can manage this within your own body.

The vagus nerve provides yet another road to satiety. After eating a meal, vagal neurons transmit information to the brain about the number of fats, particularly triglycerides and linoleic acid, that have made their way to the liver. This activates the function of the vagus nerve and sends a signal to the brain, which produces a feeling of satiety and a desire to stop eating.

Managing Blood Sugar and Insulin Levels

Insulin resistance and levels of type II diabetes are on the rise at exorbitant rates. Obesity and properly called diabesity—concurrent diabetes and obesity— are big signs of an unhealthy lifestyle. Weight problems and poor blood sugar control are signs that something in your body is working suboptimally.

Our bodies shift their balance towards the sympathetic nervous system during times of stress and release more of the adrenal stress hormones, specifically cortisol. Cortisol's primary effect is to increase blood sugar by stimulating a process called gluconeogenesis when new glucose is created from fat and protein stored in the hepatic system.

Our skeletal muscles require significant energy-forming resources to facilitate the fight-or-flight response—preferably, the fastest-acting and most easily accessible way to form cellular energy that would allow us to survive the threat. Our bodies can generate glucose rapidly and use gluconeogenesis for short-term fuel to transfer it through the bloodstream. The sympathetic nervous system swiftly shifts blood flow to the arms and leg muscles to make us extra strong and fast while shifting it away from the digestive tract and kidneys. We can then easily use our bodies to fight the threat or sprint away as quickly as possible.

For now, it is necessary to understand that nourishment can never move along this path without the vagus nerve. It starts in the pharynx, goes into the esophagus, then through the stomach, into all three parts of the small intestine, and against gravity in the ascending and transverse colon.

Managing the Activity of the Immune System

Would you drive a car with no functioning brakes? A car has the important function of moving you safely from point A to point B, and the important function of your immune system is to keep you safe from attacking your cells and proteins. And just as a car needs a system of checks and balances, like brakes, so your body's immune cells need a similar set of checks and balances.

The immune system can run out of control without its brakes and start attacking human cells, which can then lead to autoimmunity or even stop attacking tumor cells, leading to cancer. A car can be a very hazardous tool without brakes. The immune system can also be quite risky without a system to keep it in check.

Allowing Us to Create Memories

Recent research has shown that gut bacteria are essential for the growth and maturation of both the central nervous system and the enteric nervous system. As described above, the vagus nerve is heavily involved in relaying microbial information from the intestinal bacteria to the brain. This communication chain is responsible for activating the production of a protein called neurotrophic factor

(BDNF) derived from the brain. BDNF activation leads to increased neuronal connectivity, and most importantly, to memory production in the brain.

This means that it can be difficult to form new memories and create new neuronal connections without gut bacteria and a healthy functioning vagus nerve. To an even greater degree, if you have an optimally functioning vagus nerve, you are likely to be able to form larger memories and associations with the world around you.

Chapter 3:
Understanding the Vagus Nerve and Optimize your Life

I t sounds trivial, but anything we do impacts our nervous system. The trauma aftermath of the unprecedented firearms abuse and the most disturbing tales of the MeToo campaign have placed discussions of physical and mental well-being to the forefront. More than ever, people are asking what it takes to be healthy and what happens if we are attacked or stressed out.

Dr. Stephen Porges is a seasoned authority on how dire conditions ravage our bodies. He is also a promoter of instruments for restoring homeostasis and returning the nervous system to its optimum degree of harmony. His groundbreaking work began with the Polyvagal Concept, a theory he claimed, "actually offered a new vision of the universe." The way people view the autonomous nervous system has improved. In the last 100 years, our perception of the nervous system has not advanced yet, but Porges' research with the vagus nerve has turned the field on its head. When you have had simple psychology or mind-body relation lesson in the past ten years, you've undoubtedly come across this work and you're already skilled in meditation, relaxation, and yoga.

Why was it so revolutionary? Porges' Polyvagal Theory was the first to foster the recognition and interpretation of the brain mechanisms that are controlled and governed by our bodies. His principle establishes the foundation of the psychology for cognition and behavior research methods.

The vagus is the 10th and longest cranial nerve. It goes from the brain to the lower abdomen and interacts with the skin, lungs, and gastrointestinal tract. The Theories of Polyvagus understand the association between the parasympathetic regulation of certain body processes and sensory experiences of life.

Owing to the unusual connection between our lived practices and our physiological responses, the vagus nerve has become a significant index for physical and mental wellbeing. First, the vagus nerve allows the immune system to function. Inflammation can be minimized, oxytocin improved (read: enhanced desire and connectivity), along with the growth rate of stem cells. This nerve has its effect on almost everything we do. Everything we believe and do impacts the vagus nerve in our body and brain.

Defining the polyvagal principle of the nervous system

In general, the Polyvagal Hypothesis explains the reaction of our nervous system to threats or dangers in three hierarchical systems:

1. A "safe" zone: we feel confident and don't instantly feel challenged. The ventral vagal complex, a brain stem region that controls the heart and the striped muscles of the face and head, reinforces these feelings of health.

2. Fight-or-flight: we feel an activation if stressors occur in our life or atmosphere like traveling onto a plane or experiencing an unwanted noise. The sympathetic nervous system promotes this sense of security.

3. Complete immobilization: what does Dr. Porges liken to the full shutdown arising from the brainstem nucleus known as the vagus

dorsal nucleus. When we completely freeze, suffer extreme or persistent traumatic conditions such as sexual abuse and murder, our biology indicates that we are undergoing such danger to decrease metabolic production. When you feel "numb" or "frozen," like those with PTSD, the driver's seat is our dorsal vagal mechanism, and we behave like a mouse in a cat's jaws.

And what precisely does this explosion of brain and body shifts count as a stressor? Dr. Porges suggests that it may cause autoimmunity and other body disorders such as fibromyalgia, dysautonomia, and irritable bowel syndrome, better known as the "condition of protection nervous system."

Autoimmune Disease and the Nervous System

The sad fact is that we are often out of step with our nervous system. We do dumb stuff like miss meals or scarf down fast food with no concern for nutrition and how everything from memory to our energy level is impacted. Dr. Porges suggests that autoimmunity and other physical disorders — such as fibromyalgia and dysautonomia — may best be classed as "the protective nervous system." By holding our nervous system out of the way of persistent combat, we hopefully have improved safety.

It makes sense that the emergence of "invisible diseases" is correlated with the vagus and the capacity of the body (or lack thereof) to control taxing assaults that are biologically closing us. The strength of Polyvagal's hypothesis is that it provides a structure to understand more how our nervous systems should be controlled and sustained in an environment that advances at the pace of light.

Learning How to Listen to the Body

Dr. Porges showed how our culture tries to accept what our bodies are attempting to teach. Many of us have never been shown how to return to a healthy state when we feel overwhelmed or out of control. Where to begin?

"I'd agree it is a really stressful environment in which we live," Dr. Porges says. "It's not just taxing on social and mental systems; it's always challenging on our bodies. We may fulfil these standards, but we do need time to enable our bodies and minds to be healthy and comfortable. We need recovery periods, and we should start developing resilience with these recovery times. Our nervous system has evolved to perform effectively by going in and out of protection to adapt to demands and recover from demands."

Dr Porges' research influenced his everyday activities and mode of communication. When Dr. Porges grew up, he was a keen athlete and clarinetist — both at the college level. Those experiences became the basis for a revolutionary hypothesis, which allowed him to explore his ability to transcend "dustbowl empiricism" and enkindle his curiosity about the relationship between mind and body.

"The object is everything. Our engine keeps us healthy," he notes. "I did not originally know that remaining relaxed and calming has the potential to reduce negative behaviors. It was obvious to me that kindness and stopping actions would alter state-dependent behavior." Anything can significantly influence our autonomous nervous system, from social actions to internal emotions.

If you feel out of contact with your body and want to function more in tune with the nervous system, Dr. Porges has the following suggestions:

Extend the Duration of Your Exhale

Conscious breathing is the way to start. Use air as an anchor and concentrate on it while you feel anxious or exhausted. Deep exhalation facilitates the supremacy of the parasympathetic organ, which will help to return the body to a stable comfort condition. The enhanced vagal impact slows our pulse, a pace that has a soothing effect as we extend our exhalation. When nervous or experiencing a panic situation, our normal response is to take quick, shallow breaths that raise the heart rate, making you feel less rooted and more excited.

Practices such as meditation and pranayama yoga have vagotropic results that slow down and boost the heart's pumping of blood. The calming reflex by mind-body activities, such as transcendental therapy and praying, are ideal strategies to minimize the release of carbon dioxide and to slow down the body. Continuing the exhale for 2-4 seconds longer than normal would create a difference. Releasing your breath makes your body let go of fear and stress.

Listen to Music and Sing with Other People

A core concept of the Polyvagic Theory is that we are firmly rooted in a relaxed state thanks to the specific (i.e., ventral) vagal pathway, which originates in the brain stem region that controls the striated facial and facial muscles involved in listening, vocalizing and speaking. The mechanism helps humans and other primates to be social, according to Dr. Porges. "Art is modifying many channels through performing and listening." When you jamming to a favorite album, you recognize how easily music and singing can alter your mood. Of note, Tibetan lamas retain elevated rates of carbon dioxide as exhalation is prolonged while singing. Socializing also play a significant part in maintaining the health of our nervous system.

Porges invented the word "neuroception" to explain how our neuronal pathways differentiate circumstances and individuals from healthy to risky without consciousness. Protection neuroception is required before social interaction allows for social bonds. "A perceptual understanding of signals allows our biology to take on an entirely different process that occurs at a point beyond our consciousness."

"We need some social contact," he notes. "We exist in a fragmented, interactive environment, but we crave for social contact in our nervous system." If we are at rest (establishing the ventral vagal path), we are relaxed, responsive to communication, and can adapt.

Bring Awareness to Your Posture and Stand Up

"Standing up affects our alertness and causes blood pressure adjustments," says Dr. Porges. You may wonder why body coordination and stance are stressed during some yoga and meditation courses. "Ground" is a common concept in mind-body activities that implies enabling the diaphragm to be fully exhaled and relaxed. Playing and sitting in front of a computer or riding in a car for lengthy stretches may times to take a closer look at your sitting.

Really Listen to Your Body

You will alter your perception and energy by simply changing your position. You activate the parasympathetic nervous system by preserving proper posture during lengthy exhalation (the way the body relaxes). Although you will think it's too easy just to let gravity do its thing, it takes continuous practice to keep an isometric posture to strengthen your heart and help you relax through any exercise.

Chapter 4:
The Benefits of the Vagus Nerve

The vagus nerve provides nerve pathways to the pharynx (throat), larynx (voice box), trachea (windpipe), lungs, heart, thoracic, and intestinal tract as well as the transverse part of the colon. The vagus nerve brings sensory data back to the brain from the ear, tongue, pharynx, and larynx.

The vagus nerve as a cranial nerve originates from the medulla oblongata, a part of the brain stem, and extends all the way down from the brain stem to the colon. Total disruption of the vagus nerve induces a characteristic syndrome where the soft palate droops over the side where the damage occurred, along with an impaired the gag reflex.

The voice is hoarse and nasal, and the vocal cord on that side becomes immobile. The outcome is trouble swallowing (dysphagia) and talking (dysphonia). The vagus nerve has vital branches, for instance, recurrent laryngeal nerve stimulation.

Some cranial nerves deliver data to the senses (such as sight or touch) and to the brain (sensory) plus a few control muscles (engine). Peripheral nerves have both sensory and motor functions. In short, the vagus nerve controls many structures and organs, for example, the larynx (voice box), lungs, heart and gastrointestinal tract.

The vagus nerve is one of the 12 pairs of cardiovascular nerves that arise in the brain and is a part of the autonomic nervous system that controls involuntary body functions. The nerve passes through the throat as it travels between the torso and abdomen as well as the lower portion of the brain. It's linked to motor capabilities inside the voice box, diaphragm, heart and stomach and the sensory functions of the tongue and ears. It's linked to both the sensory and motor functions in the uterus and stomach.

As a mode of therapy, Vagus Nerve Stimulation (VNS) sends a regular, gentle stimulation of electric energy into the brain through the vagus nerve via a system that acts much like a pacemaker. There's no physical engagement of the brain in this operation, and patients can't generally feel the stimulation. It's necessary to remember that VNS is a therapy restricted to people with epilepsy or treatment-resistant depression.

People with any of the following might be proper candidates for VNS:

- Requiring other concurrent kinds of brain stimulation

- Heart arrhythmias or other cardiovascular problems

- Dysautonomias (the irregular functioning of the autonomic nervous system)

- autoimmune ailments or ailments (shortness of breath, asthma, etc.)

- Ulcers (gastric, esophageal, etc.)

- Vasovagal syncope (fainting)

- Pre-existing hoarseness

VNS implantation is performed by a neurosurgeon. It takes approximately 45-90 minutes with the individual commonly under anesthesia and done on an inpatient basis. Like most operations, there's a small risk of infection. Other dangers of VNS include pain or inflammation at the incision site, injury to nerves and nerve constriction. The process requires two small incisions. The very first one is left on the top left side of their torso where the pulse generator is implanted. Another incision is made directly across the left side of the neck within a crease of the skin. This is where the lean, flexible wires that link the pulse generator to the vagus nerve are added.

The implant or device is a flat, round piece of metal that measures about an inch and a half (4 centimeters) around and 10-13 mm thick, based on the version used. Newer versions might be marginally smaller. The stimulator includes a battery that could last from 1 to 15 years. After the battery is reduced, the stimulator is substituted using a less invasive procedure that requires opening the chest implants.

The stimulator is commonly triggered two to four months following implantation, although in some situations, it might be triggered in the operating room at the time of implantation. The neurologist uses a stimulator with a tiny handheld PC, programming applications and a programming wand. The potency and length of the electric impulses are all programmed.

The quantity of stimulation varies. However, it is generally initiated at a minimal level and gradually increases to a suitable amount for the person. The system runs constantly and can be programmed to switch on and off for certain amounts of time: for instance, 30 minutes and 5 minutes.

Patients are provided with a handheld magnet to maintain the stimulator at home (triggered by the doctor to a magnet). After the magnet is placed over the heartbeat via a website, additional stimulation is sent irrespective of the treatment program. Holding the magnet over the pulse generator turns off the stimulation, eliminating its ability to restart the stimulation. All of these maneuvers performed with the magnet could be accomplished by the individual, family, caregivers, or friends.

Why the Vagus Nerve is vital

Derived from the Latin term vagus, "to roam," the vagus nerve holds true to its title. From its origins in the cerebellum and brainstem, it winds through the entire body, and branches to innervate all the important organs:

- Pharynx
- Larynx
- Heart
- Esophagus
- Gut
- Small intestine
- Large intestine around the splenic flexure

This long reach results in the nerve playing a part in taste, swallowing, speech, heartbeat, digestion, and excretion. It functions as an irreplaceable member of the autonomic nervous system, or PNS, that is connected with bodily actions categorized as "rest and digest."

As its title suggests, the PNS specializes in calming down the body and digesting foods along with renewing the body's power source, among other purposes. To make this happen, the vagus nerve communicates with its related organs by discharging a neurotransmitter known as acetylcholine that helps alleviate blood pressure regulation, blood sugar equilibrium, heart rate, taste, digestion, breathing, and talking perspiration and kidney function, bile discharge, saliva secretion, and female fertility, and climaxes.

Hormones through the entire body also participate. Insulin reduces glucose release from the liver to invigorate the vagus nerve, whereas the thyroid gland, T3, stimulates the nerve to boost appetite and the creation of ghrelin.

Vagus nerve work is crucial to the launch of oxytocin, testosterone, and vasoactive intestinal peptide. The creation of growth hormone-releasing hormone, GHRH, and also the stimulation of adrenal hormone such as converting vitamin D3 into active vitamin D are given impetus

How the Vagus Nerve Impacts Mental and Physical Health

Even though the vagus impacts organs in the central nervous system, or CNS, made up of the spinal cord and the brain, it's very important to remember that it is suspended at the brainstem and cerebellum. Optimal features, or "large vagal tone indicator," are related to strong social interactions, positive feelings, and improved physical health. People with a reduced vagal tone indicator encounter depression, heart attacks, solitude, negative emotions, and even stroke.

Gut and brain health influence one another, and the vagus nerve is the connection between them. The vagal tone indicator is considered the human body's "gut feeling" which goes straight to the brain and generates a feedback loop of greater positivity or even more negativity.

Emerging studies suggest that the vagal tone indicator is set by signals discharged from the immune system, known as cytokines. Research is underway to understand how stimulating the vagus nerve delivers the capacity for healing inflammatory conditions, such as rheumatoid arthritis, even without pharmaceutical medications.

Advantages and the Truth About the Vagus Nerve

1. The vagus nerve averts inflammation. A certain quantity of inflammation following illness or injury is ordinary. However, an overabundance is connected to many diseases and ailments, from sepsis to the autoimmune disease rheumatoid arthritis. The vagus nerve works a huge system of fibers that act like spies around your organs. If they receive a sign of the incipient inflammation of cytokines or a chemical called tumor necrosis factor (TNF), they alarms the brain and pull out anti-inflammatory receptors that modulate the body's immune reaction.

2. It makes it possible to make memories. Stimulating the vagus nerves augments memory. This activity distributes the neurotransmitter norepinephrine to the amygdala. Associated studies have been performed in humans, indicating promising treatments for ailments, including Alzheimer's disease. 3. It makes it possible to breathe. Even the neurotransmitter acetylcholine, from the vagus nerve, advises the lungs. It is one reason why Botox - a frequently used cosmetically - may be potentially harmful since it disrupts acetylcholine creation. It's possible, however, to also excite your vagus nerve by performing abdominal breathing or holding your breath for four to eight counts.

4. It is intimately involved with your own heart. The vagus nerve

controls the management of the heartbeat via electric impulses to technical muscle tissues - the heart's natural pacemaker - at the right atrium, where acetylcholine release slows down the heartbeat.

By measuring the period between your personal heartbeats on a graph, physicians can decide your heart rate variability or HRV. This information provides clues regarding the durability of your heart and the needed amount of vagus nerve stimulation.

5. It starts your system's comfort response. Whenever your ever-vigilant sympathetic nervous system pops up, the flight or fight responses messages the stress hormone adrenaline and cortisol in your body. That's when the vagus nerve tells the human system to chill out by releasing acetylcholine. The vagus nerve's tendrils stretch to a lot of organs, behaving like fiber-optic wires sending directions to release proteins and enzymes such as prolactin, vasopressin, and oxytocin, which calm you down. Individuals with a powerful vagus reaction are inclined to recover more rapidly following anxiety, trauma, or disease.

6. It contrasts between your stomach and your brain. Your gut employs the vagus nerve like a walkie-talkie to inform your brain how you are feeling through electrical impulses known as "action potentials." Your gut feelings are extremely real.

7. Too much stimulation is the usual cause of fainting. Should you shake or get queasy at the sight of blood or while obtaining a flu shot, you are not weak. You are experiencing "vagal syncope." Your entire body reacts to pressure, overstimulating the vagus nerve, thus causing the blood pressure and heart rate to fall. During intense syncope, blood circulation is limited to the brain, and you lose

consciousness. But the majority of the time, you simply need to lie or sit down for the symptoms to subside.

8. The electrical stimulation of the vagus nerve decreases inflammation and might inhibit it completely. Neurosurgeon Kevin Tracey was that the first to demonstrate that stimulating the vagus nerve can considerably reduce inflammation. Outcomes on rats were successful, and he replicated the experimentation in people with magnificent results. The development of enhancements to stimulate the vagus nerve through digital implants revealed a radical reduction, and sometimes even remission, in rheumatoid arthritis, a condition with no known treatment, often requiring medications.

9. Vagus nerve stimulation has brought in a new area of medicine. Spurred on by the achievement of vagal nerve stimulation to treat swelling and epilepsy, a new area of health study called bioelectronics could be the future of medicine. Using implants that provide electrical impulses to various body components, scientists and physicians hope to take care of many illnesses with fewer drugs and fewer unwanted side effects.

VNS is not a cure for everything. But a lot of men and women who experience VNS undergo a substantial (greater than 50 percent) decrease in the incidence of epileptic seizures, in addition to a decline in seizure severity. This can considerably enhance the standard of life for those who have epilepsy.

Chapter 5:
Vagus Nerve Dysfunction

One among all the things that most people don't recognize about the vagus nerve is that it is not easy to tell when it's malfunctioning. Indeed, many people appear to be perfectly healthy on the surface but are actually suffering from a malfunctioning vagus nerve system.

This is mainly because the symptoms are psychological in some cases while physical in others. Given that the vagus nerve plays such a central role in the nervous system, it can be difficult to isolate the pain or symptoms of a disease from the ones indicating a dysfunction.

You're going to learn how to spot whether you're suffering from any of the telltale symptoms and what you can do about it. Keep in mind that it will seem as if these symptoms are related to other injuries or diseases, but the underlying cause of the disease could very well be vagus nerve dysfunction.

Chronic Nausea

I have personal experience with this. Following an accident, there was a period of a few months when I experienced intense nausea, and mealtimes became a chore. Of course, there was nothing physically wrong with my digestive system, and I hadn't contracted an eating disorder.

I just felt like puking after meals or sometimes even when smelling food. Chronic nausea will affect your appetite, as you can imagine, placing your body under further stress. The vagus nerve innervates the stomach, throat, gut, liver, mouth and brain, and it should not be surprising that your entire body will revolt against food or nutrition of any kind following trauma.

Weight Loss

If you're not going to eat thanks to constant feelings of nausea, you cannot expect your body to maintain its regular weight. I happened to lose close to 10 lbs. over three weeks following my discharge from the hospital. At first, I assumed this was merely due to inactivity, but it was connected to the lack of food intake. Being ignorant of the vagus nerve's function, I managed to ingest liquid calories in a bid to shove something down, but the nausea never went away until I began addressing the real problem.

Weight Gain

While weight loss is common, weight gain is eminently possible as well. Some people don't experience nausea but rather intense feelings of stress and anxiety. Eating is a common way for some to deal with such a situation, and the result is a steady increase in weight over time.

While weight loss happens overnight, weight gain of this kind takes time due to a surplus of calories building up. Watch out for any odd cravings you might have or a complete inability to deny yourself sugary foods the moment you get stressed or have to deal with a tough situation.

Irregular Heart Beat

Bradycardia is when your heart begins to beat at a rate lower than normal. Your blood pressure decreases drastically, and you have a problem with staying conscious. Bradycardia doesn't have to be provoked by physical activity of any kind. You could be going about your day doing normal things, and all of a sudden, dizziness and lightheadedness take over. You will also experience a shortness of breath in such moments.

Tachycardia is at the other extreme where your heart will start beating faster than normal. It is a scary experience since you're not going to lose consciousness when this happens, and you will feel as if your heart wants to burst out of your chest. This is what effectively happens during heart attacks, and you should immediately consult a medical professional.

IBS

Irritable bowel syndrome is a condition my wife experienced when she had a bout with vagus nerve malfunction. The reasons for IBS manifesting are not exactly known, but it is clear that vagus nerve malfunction has something to do with it. Constant bloating and an inability to digest food is a hallmark of IBS.

On the surface, it indicates a lack of good gut bacteria needed to break down food properly. However, as long as you're not consuming food that actively destroys these probiotic bacteria, they should replenish themselves (Haas, 2018). Constant IBS indicates a state of stress and dorsal or sympathetic activation.

Depression

As mentioned earlier, gut health and depression are linked (Haas,

2018). Add a general feeling of discomfort and inadequacy to poor gut health, and you're looking at a situation perfect for the formation of depression.

Anxiety

Anxiety goes hand in hand with depression and might make itself known first. You'll always be looking for something bad to happen, and even the smallest issue will reinforce the fact that things are bad for you at this moment.

Chronic Inflammation

The ventral vagus circuit is the one responsible for calming your body down, and it is the one that prioritizes rest and repair. As long as this is being overridden by the other two circuits, you're not going to recover. This is pretty much what was happening with my wife in increasing degrees as she first set aside her own needs to take care of me and fell sick herself.

At first, it was tough for her to understand the link between her feelings of anxiety about the future and her constant pain. Her anxiety only served to activate her dorsal circuit, and as a result, she couldn't help but simply give in to the situation she was facing. Because of this, her body was constantly stressed and never got a chance to heal or relax. Thus, inflammation was always around since nothing was ever being repaired by her body.

Constant Fatigue

Picture this: you're not eating well thanks to nausea and your brain is telling you that everything is going wrong; the best thing to do is simply curl into a ball and accept what comes. You're unlikely to have a lot of energy to do anything but give in to this feeling.

If fatigue has been your constant companion, this is a blaring sign that your vagus nerve is malfunctioning, and you're activating the circuits that do not help your well-being.

Heartburn

This is linked to digestive problems. Combined with the feelings of nausea, this can be a double whammy since not only do you feel the need to puke after eating, but you'll also suffer from heartburn thanks to your food not being digested well. Your body is not prioritizing your digestion enough, and food simply isn't being broken down properly.

The Next Steps to Take

While these symptoms are not serious as one-time occurrences, if you observe one of them occurring for over a week or even a combination of them for the same period of time, make a list and call your doctor immediately. As I mentioned, it helps to seek a professional who has knowledge of polyvagal theory.

Either way, don't delay your consultation for too long since this could cause you to become dehydrated or lose weight at an even more alarming rate. A polyvagal issue or not, you need to prioritize visiting a doctor as soon as possible. Be prepared to reply to the questions about your medical (history) and let your doctor know of any past trauma you've suffered or any history of disease.

In my wife's and my experiences, an initial medical examination ensued. This involved the usual poking and prodding with a stethoscope followed by even more questions. It can be tough for your doctor to pinpoint the exact reasons for your discomfort and get to the main reason for the problem.

If most of your problems are related to digestion, you will likely undergo an endoscopy or an x-ray examination. X-rays are a non-invasive procedure, and it is likely that your doctor will opt for this method first to detect any blockages in your stomach. An endoscopy involves a tube being inserted down your digestive tract with a camera attached to it.

This procedure is as unpleasant as it sounds, but it does give your doctor a good view of what is happening within you. In addition to this, a procedure called an esophageal manometry test might be conducted on you. This measures your stomach's contraction rate and involves a tube being stuck up your nose and left in for 15 minutes.

A more advanced test that is carried out if you repeatedly complain of digestive symptoms is a gastric emptying study. In this, you'll eat a lightly irradiated piece of food which will allow your doctor to track how fast your body digests it. Generally speaking, if the food is still in your stomach after an hour and a half, this points to some form of digestive disorder.

An ultrasound can also be used to detect any blockages in your gut. The test that is conducted as a last resort if your doctor is unable to detect anything is an electrogastrogram. In this test, a couple of electrodes will be placed outside your belly, and your doctor will listen to your stomach for an hour or so.

Vagal Tone

Vagal tone refers to the baseline activity of the vagus nerve, specifically the ventral system (Haas, 2018). Measuring vagal tone is not a straightforward task, but invasive and noninvasive procedures do exist. Often, the easiest way to measure vagal tone is to measure bodily processes that are affected by it.

One of the most commonly measured functions is the heart rate. Generally speaking, in human beings, a base heart rate between 55-100 beats per minute is considered healthy. Any variation from this range is likely to be a cause of concern. More than the resting heart rate, it is the heart rate's variability that is important.

When we breathe in, our heart rates increase and with every breath out; it slows down just a little bit. The difference between the heart rate on exhalation and inhalation is called the heart rate's variability. A lower degree of variability indicates faster vagal response and a higher tone.

A low vagal tone often results in conditions such as chronic inflammation since the vagus nerve is the one that is responsible for switching the body's immune system back on and restoring its healing abilities. In people with low vagal tones, this doesn't happen, and thus inflammation persists.

Vagal tone doesn't just affect your physical functions but emotional ones as well. A research study published in 1994 found that the physiological regulation of emotions was directly affected by vagal tone (Haas, 2018).

The study determined this by measuring the amount of cortisol that was present in the bloodstream of their subjects. As a bit of a background, cortisol is a hormone that is associated with stress and is a by-product of the stress response. Continuously high levels of cortisol in the bloodstream lead to conditions such as IBS.

It isn't cortisol itself that causes this but the malfunctioning vagus nerve that precipitates such a condition. In this particular study, researchers measured emotional regulation in the brain by measuring both cortisol and monitoring brain activity via an EEG test. EEG stands for Electroencephalography and involves electrodes being placed on the subject's scalp.

EEG activity can be correlated to emotional activity within the brain, and researchers can thus match increased activity with baseline data. Prior research has indicated that the expression of emotion and the ability to practice emotional self-regulation is closely associated with vagal tones. In other words, the higher the vagal tone is, the quicker the subject in question is able to return to a healthy state of being (a ventral state).

Chapter 6:
What Happens to Your Digestive Tract When You Don't Take Care of the Vagus Nerve

Our vagus nerve is stimulated both involuntarily and voluntarily. If it's not stimulated properly, many problems can arise because your vagus nerve affects the rest of the body.

It Can Affect Your Appetite

Have you eaten only a tiny amount of food and realized you're full? That's a sign of your vagus nerve at work. It controls all communication up and down the body, taking care of hunger and the signals of being full. When you've eaten enough, the signal for satisfaction goes all the way up to your brain, telling it that you're not hungry anymore after eating a meal.

There are also different neurotransmitters inside our stomach, like serotonin and ghrelin that send feelings of hunger and fullness to the vagus nerve within the brain. As such, your vagus nerve controls all perceptions of hunger, mood and stress levels and the information regarding the inflammatory response in the body. The signals go from the brain toward the gut after you digest food, and the digestive enzymes are all affected.

Your vagus nerve also works on pushing food out of your body, which is another way of saying it controls how much you defecate and whether or not you're suffering from diarrhea or constipation.

This important pathway controls many factors, including your health and weight. So what happens if you don't take care of your vagus nerve?

Fullness Signals

The vagus nerve isn't properly working when you're obese and isn't as sensitive to the neurotransmitters for fullness. This means you end up overeating and not getting enough exercise, causing more weight gain and obesity. However, there are regimens that can change how your vagus nerve reacts to everything.

It takes a huge amount of food to tell your brain that you're full when you're obese. It also doesn't have a very strong fullness signal, so even if you do tell the brain you're full, the vagus nerve isn't working as strongly as it should. If your vagus nerve is stimulated properly, it turns on these fullness signals in both animals and in humans. So, when if turn the signals on, you'll eat a lot less, lose weight, and feel fuller.

Irritable Bowel Syndrome

IBS (Irritable bowel syndrome) happens when you have abdominal pain from the digestive movements, but it can be lessened or cured with the help of your vagus nerve. If your vagus nerve is stimulated, it can help remove waste from your body and reduce pain. Vagal tone controls the motility of your body and helps with gastrointestinal pain, especially that associated with dyspepsia and Irritable Bowel Syndrome.

Insulin Resistance

Insulin resistance is a diabetic condition in which you need more insulin to help break down the body's sugars. For those with diabetes or prediabetes, this can be a problem because it takes much more insulin to reduce blood sugar levels, and they tend to increase.

Your vagus nerve has some authority over your pancreas too, where you secrete insulin to help break down glucose molecules. It dulls the vagus nerve when you're not eating correctly, which affects insulin performance in the body. It takes a whole lot of insulin to break it down, which is why those with diabetes need medication to help reduce this.

Inflammation factors also play their part. When you're not taking care of the vagus nerve and instead are just eating whatever you want, insulin resistance especially happens. When you stimulate the vagus nerve properly, you'll be able to reduce blood glucose and insulin levels.

Gut-Brain Connection

Your vagus nerve directly connects your gut and brain. However, something else is involved stimulating your gut and brain together to counteract hunger and help move everything around. This is called Lactobacillus reuteri, also known as L. reuteri. It's a bacterium that's a part of your microbiome, which helps stimulate food breakdown as you ingest it.

The L. reuteri do this job by giving your brain the signal that, hey, there's food here. This is your gut health working, and it reduces inflammation within the body.

This bacterium helps the neurotransmitters calm your gut and make it, so your body is properly digesting food. It also secretes oxytocin and dopamine, which reduces pain and stimulates blood flow. Dopamine primarily is used in this way.

If the vagus nerve isn't appropriately stimulated, these neurotransmitters won't work, and your body cannot fight off the inflammation coming from your stomach acids, the foods you eat, and the like. This causes a "leaky gut," a permeability of the intestines where the toxins and bacteria tend to "leak" through the intestine walls.

Leaky Gut

Your vagus nerve makes sure that harmful substances are properly broken down through neurotransmitters' function. It also helps the peristalsis of the body. Your digestive tract aids this to protect the body from harmful bacteria and substances. Your intestinal walls are vitally barriers that control the bloodstream and everything brought to the organs. The small gaps in your intestinal wall permit a variety of nutrients to be delivered while also blocking the passage of harmful substances. Intestinal permeability is fundamentally the reason why these substances easily go through the intestinal wall.

When these junctions become loose, it essentially affects how permeable the gut becomes, allowing toxins and bacteria to enter the bloodstream. Your vagus nerve manages this inflammatory response and helps keep everything tight. If the vagus nerve isn't appropriately stimulated, the "leaky" gut happens, and uncontrolled and widespread inflammation occurs within your body, causing autoimmune conditions to take root and fester. For example, bloating, sensitivities, digestive issues, skin problems, and fatigue may occur due to this.

If your vagus nerve is adequately stimulated and working properly, it can reduce the inflammatory response, thus reducing inflammation in the body. We'll go into further detail on inflammation, but understand that your gut isn't just a place where food is digested. It's also a location where a lot happens that isn't fun for anyone.

Taking Care of the Vagus Nerve Through Nutrition

When you find ways of improving your vagus nerve, you are addressing what you're putting into your body. When you have a "cafeteria diet," which involves lots of fats and carbs, it reduces the vagus nerve's sensitivity. However, eating a low-carb diet a bit higher in fat can help. There are ways to stimulate the vagus nerve through a variety of tools, but it's a little more complex than you'd think.

A lousy regimen just makes you feel gross, and part of it is because your vagus nerve isn't being correctly stimulated. A good regimen helps to counteract these problems, maybe even restoring them. We'll highlight what you can do to help properly stimulate the vagus nerve, but being mindful of what you eat is very important. It can help reduce the possibility of leaky gut and also with your microbiome.

It is pertinent to focus on the bacteria within the body. Whether through the foods you eat or through supplements, probiotics are essential for vagus nerve health. The right foods will change the body. You'll have a healthier body with the proper stimulation and the right bacteria and fewer instances of leaky gut or other intestinal issues.

Your brain and gut are connected, as stated, if only through this nerve. Understand that what you put into your body plays a significant role in how your vagal tone improves and how you respond to the world around you. Let's talk about inflammation and how your vagus nerve controls it.

Treatment-resistant Depression

Studies suggested a potential decrease in the symptoms of depression in patients who had the system implanted for seizure control shortly after the FDA approved VNS as a seizure treatment. It is suspected that VNS acts like electroconvulsive therapy by using

electricity to control the output of brain chemicals called

neurotransmitters.

VNS should not be performed in patients with any of the following:

- Acute suicidal thoughts or behavior

- History of psychotic, psychotic, or delusional disorders

- History of fast cycling bipolar disorder

Gastroparesis

Research findings have shown a direct link between gastroparesis and vagus nerve damage. It's a condition that affects the involuntary contraction of the digestive system severely. As mentioned, the vagus nerve, in conjunction with ANS, facilitates the parasympathetic functions of the body. Some of the parasympathetic functions include the involuntary contraction of the digestive system. In simple terms, when you suffer from a damaged vagus nerve, you may never enjoy the parasympathetic actions of defecation. The stomach does not empty properly, and this leads to a continuous pile up of dirt before. Some of the common symptoms of this condition include:

• Nausea or vomiting: This can be much worse and severe. With gastroparesis, the patient is unable to digest most of the food eaten. This leads to nausea and vomiting long hours after eating. In normal vomiting situations, a person just vomits a few minutes after eating. However, in advanced cases of gastroparesis, the afflicted is likely to vomit after several hours of waiting.

• Loss of appetite: Most people who suffer from gastroparesis often eat a little food because they constantly lack an appetite. This condition makes a person feel full even when hungry. Patients However, there are other conditions that may lead to a lack of appetite. If you suspect you are suffering from a lack of appetite, investigate all the possible causes. A doctor can test you for vagus nerve dysfunction.

• Acid reflux: Acid refluxes will occur. However, with gastroparesis, they will be much more severe and recurrent.

• Abdominal pain or bloating: The other direct symptom of gastroparesis is bloating and abdominal pain. The vagus nerve spreads to the lower abdomen, having an influence on your excretory and sexual organs. This means that any damage to the nerve may directly affect your sexual or digestive health. Such conditions will often lead to abdominal pain.

• Unexplained weight loss: There are several reasons why a person suffering from gastroparesis may lose weight. First, such individuals do not eat as much as they should, and the body is denied some of its essential vitamins. Further, the body does not fully digest the food consumed. In most cases, the food leaves through vomiting, often leading to a loss of weight in most patients.

This is a distinctive observation in the severe stage of vagus nerve damage. In the early symptoms, the patient may experience digestive complications, but they are not affecting personal weight. In essence, those who suffer from the early stages of vagus nerve damage still have a choice to make on the types of foods they want to eat. They may still eat without vomiting. However, in the stage where gastroparesis develops, it is almost impossible to manage the effects associated with eating.

Chapter 7:
The Vagus Nerve Reduction of Various Inflammations

Inflammation is the body's defense against injury or invasion. The most familiar form of inflammation is acute inflammation. You've experienced this when you stubbed your toe. It is characterized by five signs: redness, swelling, warmth, pain, and mobility loss if the injury is near a joint. These are all strategies that your immune system is using to protect you. In the proper context, they are all good.

Acute Inflammation

When an injury first occurs, affected cells in the immediate area release chemicals to alert the immune response. Blood rushes to the wound's site, where the capillaries dilate to allow white blood cells through the capillary lining. The infantry unit of white blood cells floods into the offending area. They will search for invaders to destroy before an infection can set in. The redness and swelling are caused by the increase in blood to the area. The heat is caused by the blood also because it quickly came from deeper within your body, where the core temperature is typically warmer than your outer skin.

Mobility loss from the excess blood happens if there's less room for your joints to move. When a decrease in mobility does occur, it makes you less likely to worsen the injury by immobilizing the area, similar to a natural splint. Pain occurs if there are pain receptors in the location of the damage, but it serves a function also. It forces you to protect and treat the area differently, allowing it the time and space to heal. If you don't clean the wound properly, unfriendly microorganisms are given access to your body through the skin's opening. A skirmish between the microorganisms and your white blood cells will follow. This battle may result in pus that collects at the site of the action, evidence of the casualties of war.

If the injury is internal, the body's response is similar but perhaps less noticeable. Blood will still rush to the area. The capillaries will again dilate to release the army of white blood cells for their search and destroy mission. This rush of blood causes swelling and perhaps a loss of mobility, depending upon the degree of swelling, pain, and location. Heat, unless the infection has set in, isn't an issue because internal injuries are already at the core body temperature. And the pain may or may not occur, depending on whether there are any pain receptors in the area of concern.

Chronic Inflammation

Whether the injury or invasion is internal or external, the acute immune response's effects will last anytime between hours to several days, depending on the severity of the issue. On the other hand, chronic inflammation is a similar response, but its signs may be less noticeable. You may experience fatigue, a low-grade fever, random rashes, and dull pain in the chest or abdomen without realizing why.

These effects last much longer, though, and can harm the otherwise healthy surrounding tissue over time. You may even come to a point wherein you are so accustomed to the fatigue, dull pain, and skin irritations that you are barely even aware of them. It becomes your usual mode of operation. This gradual demise is how chronic inflammation can take over your life. Recent studies implicate chronic inflammation as the leading suspect for a wide range of severe diseases.

There are a few causes of chronic inflammation. The most obvious is if it is left untreated. A horrifying yet real example of this was in the news a few years ago when a surgeon accidentally left an instrument in the patient's body before sewing it up. The patient experienced unexplainable pain, random bouts of fever, and debilitating fatigue for years before an X-ray for an unrelated exam discovered the offending forceps. Once the forceps were removed and the lawsuit was underway, the patient had a full recovery.

Another, more frequent, cause of chronic inflammation is an autoimmune disorder. Numerous studies have linked the vagus nerve to this cause of chronic inflammation. Andersson and Tracey in 2012, Tracey in 2016, and Pavlov and Tracey in 2017 have described a response reflex that triggers the vagus nerve to suppress or release signals that call for the immune response army. However, doctors don't thoroughly understand why, sometimes, the inflammatory reflex goes awry. When this happens, "friendly fire" is the result. The body attacks itself, leading to a plethora of conditions known as a chronic disease.

Crohn's disease, rheumatoid arthritis, diabetes, obesity, heart disease, asthma, and even Alzheimer's are just some of the conditions that can be linked to chronic inflammation. During the 2020 coronavirus pandemic, the two most significant risk factors for predicting who would suffer the most or die were age and pre-existing chronic diseases. All of those pre-existing diseases are caused by inflammation. Even age, although certainly not caused by inflammation, is amplified by inflammation.

One's regimen can be a huge factor in controlling inflammation. You should strictly avoid highly processed carbohydrates, unhealthy fats, sugar, and processed meats that can trigger an immune response. People who have spent their lives eating mostly these types of food will most definitely suffer from some inflammatory condition at some point in their lives.

Conversely, olive oil, fatty fish, berries, and green leafy vegetables can all have anti-inflammatory properties. These healthy foods should comprise the majority of your diet. People who eat such items can expect to live in relatively good health well into their old age. Supplements and spices can also help reduce inflammation. Fish oil supplements and curcumin have been associated with a reduction in inflammation, as well as ginger, garlic, and cayenne pepper.

When dietary changes aren't enough to control the inflammation, you can purchase over the counter drugs such as Advil and Aleve that are nonsteroidal anti-inflammatory drugs (NSAIDs). However, using these drugs long term has risks, such as peptic ulcer and kidney disease. If a better diet and NSAIDs don't do the trick, steroids, for which you need a prescription, can reduce inflammation and suppress the immune response. They also have long-term risks associated with them. Vision problems, high blood pressure, and osteoporosis are just a few. There are also instant side effects, such as weight gain, moodiness, and increased body hair.

Another treatment with very few risks or side effects, however, is now being explored. VNS therapy, which was used to treat epilepsy and depression, is now being studied to inhibit the vagus nerve's immune response.

Infection or injury activates the release of cytokines. Cytokines, a type of protein that signal molecules for the inflammatory response, are produced in the spleen. The vagus nerve inhibits the output in a process called the inflammatory reflex. Studies have found that targeting this reflex with a VNS device in patients with rheumatoid arthritis and Crohn's disease reduces cytokine production.

Rheumatoid Arthritis

Unlike osteoarthritis, rheumatoid arthritis is an immune response that attacks the lining of the joints, causing painful swelling, bone erosion, and joint deformity. It begins in the smaller joints such as fingers and spreads to more substantial joints such as elbows and knees. In most cases, inflammation attacks the joints on both sides of the body. In about 40% of cases, tissues other than the joints can become affected, such as the eyes, skin, heart, and lungs. Doctors don't exactly know what triggers this autoimmune disorder. They think a viral or bacterial response may cause the onset. Traditionally, doctors treat this disease with medication, but not all subjects respond to medication.

In a 2019 presentation at the Annual European Congress of Rheumatology, Dr. Mark Genovese, MD, presented the findings of a SetPoint Medical research study on VNS therapy. The study sought treatments to alleviate the symptoms of rheumatoid arthritis. He cited an earlier study that involved 17 patients with non-responsive rheumatoid arthritis who had the VNS device surgically implanted. After six weeks of daily 60-second stimulation periods, participants noticed that their symptoms significantly disappeared. Then the researchers turned the VNS device off for two weeks, and the patient's symptoms quickly began to return. Then at eight weeks, the device was turned on again, and the symptoms were reduced again.

Dr. Genovese then presented the findings of two more recent studies using a newer VNS device model. The more modern device eliminates the need for a chest incision or connecting wire. Instead, they implant the much smaller charge generator in the same location as the coils around the vagus nerve. The patient must plug in a wireless charging apparatus once a week, and the doctor can control the device settings via a smartphone app.

The first recent study he reported had just three participants. They had the new VNS model implanted and were given stimulation for one minute per day. These individuals also, very quickly, began to see an improvement in symptoms.

The second recent study involved 11 participants. The researchers fractionate the participants into three groups. One group received the new VNS model, and the researchers gave them one minute of stimulation once a day. A second group received the new VNS model, and the researchers gave them one minute of stimulation four times a day. The third group received a sham device. Like the two studies, the first group noticed a quick and significant improvement in their rheumatoid arthritis symptoms. The second group, interestingly enough, saw no improvement at all. One participant's symptoms even began increasing. There was no alternation in the symptoms of the sham group.

Crohn's Disease

Crohn's disease is an illness that causes inflammation in the colon and latter part of the small intestines, with symptoms that include fatigue, abdominal pain, diarrhea, and weight loss. It can be debilitating and painful and may even lead to life-threatening complications. Doctors don't fully understand what causes the disease, but they think that a viral or bacterial response triggers it. Certain stressors and foods can aggravate the symptoms.

There is no cure, but there are medications that may help reduce the symptoms in some people. But like every treatment plan, there are some whose disease is resistant to it. In other people, the side effects outweigh the benefits. More than half of the patients with Crohn's disease will need surgery to remove part of the intestines or colon. This drastic measure isn't necessarily a cure, though. Eventually, the condition may re-establish itself in the remaining parts of the intestines and colon.

A 2016 study by Bonaz et al. involved seven patients with Crohn's disease. The researchers treated them with cervical VNS. Five of the seven responded positively to the treatment, but two actually worsened. All of them reported voice alteration side effects during stimulation and coughing, pain, and labored breathing. Epilepsy and depression patients reported these same side effects.

In the May 2019 edition of Frontiers in Neuroscience, a study titled, Anti-inflammatory Effects of Abdominal Vagus Nerve Stimulation on Experimental Intestinal Inflammation, describes the findings of Payne et al. They induced an inflammatory response in rodents and treated it with VNS. They didn't use cervical VNS, however. The cervical VNS had too many off-target reactions. Besides affecting the pharynx and larynx, heart rate and breathing were also affected.

Instead, they wanted to position the VNS closer to the intestines. They devised an apparatus similar to the cervical VNS device, but they implanted it in the rodents' abdomens. After activating it, they found that nothing other than the intestines were affected. They also found that the device was successful in reducing inflammation in the intestines. They propose this to be a safe and effective treatment for Crohn's disease in humans.

Cold Therapy to Stimulate the Vagus Nerve

Ultimately, you do not have to continue to suffer from chronic, widespread inflammation. If triggering the vagus nerve through VNS works to aid inflammation relief, you should also be able to trigger the same results using methods at home that automatically tone and trigger the vagus nerve. Another such method is known as cold therapy.

When you expose your body to something drastically colder than your body, you tend to do several things: you lower the inflammation in the area, you trigger yourself to be sleepier, and you constrict your blood vessels, and in doing so, you will find that the heart rate also slows down as well. Effectively, a quick exposure to sudden cold can actually help activate your vagus nerve, triggering it to give you all its benefits.

Deciding to expose yourself to cold should always be done safely, however. Keep in mind that people can, and do, die from exposure to the cold if it is not managed well. You can get hypothermia if your body drops too low below its base temperature, and for that reason, it is critical to make sure that when engaging in any exposure to the cold, you do so responsibly. Make sure that your exposure is short and that you properly warm yourself up after.

Some choose to dive into icy lakes to trigger their own cold therapy, while others may give themselves ice baths. No matter what you do, make sure to use common sense. Do not decide to go and sleep in a pile of snow without the proper clothing. Perhaps the safest way to do cold therapy is in the comfort of your own home with a splash of cold water.

When you use cold water on your face, you trigger the same reaction. You make sure that your body responds to the sudden drop in temperature without having to expose yourself to a dangerous situation.

All you have to do is use cold water on your face. Let your faucet run as cold as possible. Splash the cold water on your face a few times to trigger your body to respond. If you want to be a bit more extreme, take a cold shower or fill your bathtub with water and ice. Ultimately, the method you choose is up to you, and so long as you chose one you can tolerate and do it regularly, you should see a decrease in inflammation.

As a bonus, if you find that your hands are particularly inflamed, the splashes of cold water with your hands may actually help make your hands feel better as well.

Chapter 8:
The Vagus Nerve and Autoimmune Disease

Autoimmune disease and the vagus nerve are as closely linked as inflammation and the vagus nerve because inflammation and autoimmune issues are intricately related—inflammation is an autoimmune response. A handful of autoimmune issues have already been tackled thus far. You have learned about arthritis and diabetes. However, there are several other autoimmune diseases that people can suffer from.

Immune disorders can go either way: they can result from an overactive immune system or an immune system that is not sufficiently active. Either way, there are issues with the body managing its own illnesses as it defense systems fail one way or the other. The end result is that some part of the body fails to engage in fighting off the illness, infection, or another trigger.

The Immune System

Through the immune system the body defends itself from illness or infection. It consists of several different types of white blood cells. There are phagocytes, which attack the bacteria or virus that have infiltrated the body and lymphocytes, another variety of white blood cells. They document the structure of the virus or bacteria, allowing the body to remember the problematic invader and prevent it from arising in the future. Both phagocytes and lymphocytes come in various forms, with each and every one acting as a specialized soldier for the job. Some are trained to do generic care, while others are more specialized. For example, B lymphocytes lock onto targets that need to be defeated before signaling that the system needs help.

The immune system works in several ways in creates three different forms of immunity. People can have what is known as innate immunity, adaptive immunity, or passive immunity. Each of these functions differently, but the result is the body having a defense against some form of the disease. Depending on which it is, people have a slightly different form of immunity with a slightly different impact.

What is Autoimmune Disease?

Autoimmune diseases are forms of disease that develop when the immune system does not function properly and, instead, becomes overactive. During periods of being overactive and running rampant, the immune system attacks the body instead of anything toxic or dangerous. This then directly damages the body, causing injury, inflammation, and suffering.

The best way to treat autoimmune disease is to find a way to slow down and reduce the immune system, and in doing so, the flare-up of the autoimmune disease should fade away, allowing for relief. Some of these autoimmune diseases will only cause problems in one area of the body, while others will impact everything, creating feelings of discomfort and suffering. Nevertheless, regardless of the harm from the autoimmune issue you are suffering from, it becomes important to ensure that the body is preserved in the best possible condition.

Some of these tendencies for creating autoimmune issues can be directly related to genetics, with studies linking them to the families, while it is believed that diet and exercise can also cause autoimmune disorders. One last topic is the hygiene hypothesis. Due to the fact that children are exposed to far fewer germs now than ever before due to immunizations becoming commonplace and the development of sanitizing cleaners that kill germs, the immune system develops a tendency to overreact. Effectively, because the immune system is not being triggered on the regular, it becomes faulty. Despite this theory, however, it is currently unknown what for sure makes people prone to disorders or why they develop.

Common Autoimmune Issues

There are over eighty autoimmune issues you could suffer from. Some of these are common, while others are practically unknown. Of the 80, 14 are relatively common. These disorders are common enough, for the most part, that if you mention them, people will have heard of them.

These 14 diseases include:

· Celiac Disease: A disease in which the immune system directly attacks the digestive system, leading to gastrointestinal sensitivity and inflammation.

· Sjögren's Syndrome: A disease in which the immune system attacks the glands within the eyes that create tears and lubrication. It is most commonly seen as dry eye and mouth.

· Addison's Disease: A disease in which the adrenal glands are unable to produce hormones at the proper rate, leading bodily malfunction.

· Hashimoto's Thyroiditis: A disease in which the thyroid does not produce enough hormones. It then leads to weight gain, struggling to tolerate the cold, goiter, and hair loss.

· Psoriatic Arthritis: A disease in which the immune system causes the skin to develop too quickly; the excess skin develops patches that become inflamed and scaly. Arthritis sometimes goes along with psoriasis, leading to joint pains and problems.

· Pernicious Anemia: A disease in which the body does not get enough protein and struggles to produce DNA effectively.

· Inflammatory Bowel Disease: A disease commonly referred to as IBD in which the immune system targets the intestinal wall. This can present in several different forms that lead to inflammation of the GI tract, leading to pain and difficulty digesting food properly.

· Autoimmune Vasculitis: A disease in which the immune system impacts the blood vessels in the body, leading to inflammation of the vessels, which then causes the veins and arteries to become more narrow, simultaneously making blood flow more difficult.

· Multiple Sclerosis: A disease in which the immune system targets the brain—particularly the myelin sheath, the part of neurons that coats the axon to bolster transmission of the impulse. As this becomes damaged, the individual's effectiveness at passing along messages becomes decreases.

· Grave's Disease: A disease in which the immune system attacks the thyroid, leading to too many hormones being produced and released into the body. This can lead to high heart rates, struggling to tolerate heat, and unexplained weight loss.

· Myasthenia Gravis: A disease in which the immune system damages the way that the brain communicates with the muscles by impacting the nerves that communicate from the mind to the body, leading to muscle weakening that seems get worse when more action is engaged in.

· Type 1 Diabetes Mellitus: A disease in which the immune system targets cells within the pancreas responsible for insulin production, causing the body to no longer process glucose effectively.

Autoimmune Disease and the Vagus Nerve

Remember, the vagus nerve directly informs the brain when there is inflammation somewhere in the body, so it can then influence just how much inflammation is allowed. However, when the vagus nerve becomes damaged, it is not capable of protecting the body from inflammation. The inflammation runs rampant, creating havoc in the body, all because the vagus nerve malfunctioned in some way.

Stop for a moment and consider all the possible implications and recognize the sheer number of people who are suffering from an autoimmune disease—upwards of 8% of the population are believed to suffer from an autoimmune disorder. Eight people of every 100 you pass are likely suffering from an autoimmune disorder or malfunctioning, and because of that, their bodies are directly attacking themselves.

Stimulation of the vagus nerve, however, has been shown to help fight inflammation, which should also help alleviate some of the autoimmune response. With the inflammation limited, the body is no longer sending cues to tackle parts of the body that did not require an actual intervention from the immune system in the first place.

Effectively, the afferent path - the path from the body to the brain - communicates to the body either a current injury or the need for the inflammation and immune response. It has been found that when the afferent nerve is blocked in some way, but the efferent pathway is free to continue as normal, the body regulates itself.

It allows for the continued communication from the brain to the body while stopping the brain from producing more hormones that encourage inflammation because it is not receiving the impulses telling the brain that inflammation is happening and needs to continue. In blocking the afferent while encouraging the efferent impulses, the body has a chance to regulate itself, and it stops producing the cytokines that will create further the inflammation responsible for the attack of the body by the immune system.

Chapter 9:
Vagus Nerve Stimulation for Epilepsy, Anxiety, and Drug Cravings

Epilepsy

Q uantum brain healing relies on a base of orthomolecular medicine including aminoacids, vitamins, minerals, herbs, botanical extracts, Chinese herbal formulas, and many alternative therapies. There is no answer that will address healing for everyone. It is key to remain open to technology when other options have not met our goals. One option often overlooked after trying nutritional therapy is Vagus Nerve Stimulation. This is a medical device that is surgically implanted. Any major medical center in the US and Europe can implant this device for a patient that qualifies.

Vagus Nerve Stimulation (VNS) involves sending a message to the brain using periodic mild electrical stimulation from the vagus nerve in the neck by a surgically implanted small medical device. There is no brain surgery involved. This stimulation or pulse is sent by a medical device similar to a pacemaker. The vagus nerve is part of the autonomic nervous system and controls involuntary body functions.

VNS may control epilepsy in cases where antiepileptic drugs are ineffective or have intolerable side effects, or neurosurgery is not appropriate for some reason. VNS is effective in stopping seizures in some patients.

The implanted medical device is a flat, round battery, and measures about the size of a silver dollar. The VNS medical device was developed by Cyberonics, Inc. The doctor determines the strength and timing of the pulses administered by the device according to each patient's individual needs. The level of electrical stimulation can be changed without additional surgery with a programming wand connected to a laptop computer.

The side effects of VNS during treatment may include hoarseness, coughing, throat pain, shortness of breath, a short and slight sensation of choking, altered voice sound, ear pain, tooth pain, and a tingling sensation in the neck. Skin irritation or infection could occur at the implantation site. VNS does not negatively impact the brain. This is major surgery and should not be considered lightly.

For those with uncontrollable epileptic seizures, it may be last option. Consider all options before giving up on controlling seizure. This is not neurosurgery and it is safer. We have been mentioning epilepsy or seizure disorder throughout this book because it was the primary disorder targeted by the vagus nerve stimulation. Furthermore, many positive benefits of vagus nerve stimulation were discovered while researchers were studying the effects of it with epilepsy.

Epilepsy is a major central nervous disorder in which brain activity becomes exceedingly abnormal, causing seizures or periods of a very unusual behavior. The nerves and neurons are firing uncontrollably, causing erratic and uncontrollable movements. A person who has epilepsy has their whole world turned upside down due to the severity of the condition and the way it takes over their life. A person will often never know when a seizure will hit, which can prevent them from doing many activities like driving. It will also inhibit their ability to go into certain professions. It is a dangerous and stressful disease to deal with.

During an epileptic episode, the sympathetic nervous system is incomplete overdrive, causing excessive and erratic movements within the nervous system. When a person is having a full-blown epileptic attack or seizure, we won't attempt the many stimulating practices discussed. Much more extreme measures will needed. However, the vagal tone can be strengthened to help avoid or reduce epileptic future attacks. The stronger the vagal tone, the better the parasympathetic response will be at inhibiting the sympathetic response. We mentioned how massaging the carotid sinus has been shown to inhibit seizure activity by stimulating the vagus nerve. If this technique works, then it is a good indication that the other methods will also work.

The overall goal is to continuously improve and strengthen the vagus nerve as much as possible. We will not be able to prevent or cure all illnesses. However, as we maintain our vagal tone, we can help to improve the functionality of the body and at least prevent or reduce many diseases. The point of vagus nerve stimulation is to keep it healthy, active, and strong so it has the ability to enhance parasympathetic activity as much as possible. When we increase our body's ability to utilize the parasympathetic response, we will reduce seizure activity effectively.

Most of the research behind vagus nerve stimulation has been to help prevent epilepsy. This suggests that it is still considered a strong therapy in inhibiting seizure activity.

Dealing with Anxiety Using Your Vagus Nerve

How often do you have to deal with anxiety in your everyday life? If you find yourself worrying too much or getting caught up in non-stopping irrational thoughts or even feeling nausea, chest pain and heart palpitations, then this book is for you.

You are about to learn a simple yet very effective technique to deal with anxiety naturally by stimulating your vagus nerve. This powerful technique can be used to relieve stress and anxiety anywhere and anytime: at home, when commuting and, of course, during those horrible work meetings.

Did you know that the FDA has approved a surgically-implanted device that is successful at treating depression by periodically stimulating the vagus nerve? But hopefully you won't need surgery. You can enjoy the benefits of vagus nerve stimulation by adopting some simple breathing techniques.

<u>Singing and diaphragmatic breathing techniques</u> strengthen this living nervous system, paying great dividends, and the best tool to achieve that is by training your breath.

<u>Breathe with your diaphragm</u>: Now it's time to put this concept into practice. The first thing you need to do is breathe using your diaphragm (abdominal breathing). This is the foundation of proper breathing and anxiety relief.

The diaphragm is your primary breathing muscle. It is belled shaped and when you inhale it patterns out (or should flatten out), acting as piston and creating vacuum in your thoracic cavity so your lungs can expand and air gets in.

On the other side it creates pressure, pushing the viscera down and out, expanding the belly. That's why good breathing practice is described as abdominal breathing or belly breathing. Nervousness can be a genuine doozy; it's outlandishly muddled, profoundly close to home, and ridiculously difficult to foresee. There are times when we think our uneasiness is behind us, that we are at long last one stage ahead, then something happens, and we are on our heels once more, battling to return to a position of harmony and quiet. We are the understudies of our uneasiness, and seeing precisely how our sensory system functions and what we can do to quiet it can be staggeringly enabling.

In any case, what does "quietening your sensory system" truly mean? Numerous individuals depict it as easing back the pulse, developing the breath, and loosening up various muscles; however, what really associates these sensations in the mind? You need to know more about the vagus nerve, the piece of the body that appears to clarify how our psyches control our bodies, how our bodies impact our brains and may give us the instruments we have to quieten them both.

Posttraumatic stress issues (PTSD) are encountered by numerous individuals. Ongoing catastrophic events, mass shootings, psychological oppressor assaults, and urban communities under attack add to the worldwide weight of PTSD, which as indicated by a recent report, influences 4–6% of the worldwide populace, despite the fact that most injuries are identified with mishaps and sexual or physical savagery. Shockingly, there is no known fix, and flow medicines are not powerful for all patients.

A PTSD psychopharmacology working group, as of late, distributed their accord proclamation calling for a quick activity to address the emergency in PTSD treatment, referring to three significant concerns. To start, just two medications (sertraline and paroxetine) are endorsed by the US FDA for the treatment of PTSD. These meds decrease the side effect's seriousness; however, they may not create a total reduction of the side effects.

The subsequent concern is identified with polypharmacy. PTSD patients are recommended prescriptions to address every one of their numerous extraordinary and assorted side effects, including nervousness, trouble dozing, sexual brokenness, wretchedness and interminable torment, while lacking exact examinations of medication communications. The high comorbidity among PTSD and fixation creates further difficulties for pharmacotherapies. The third significant concern is the absence of headway in the treatment of PTSD; no new prescriptions have been endorsed since 2001.

Drug Cravings

Addiction to any substance can make the life of an individual go topsy-turvy. From spending a fortune to deceiving one's own family, a person addicted to illegal substances will go to any extent. But how does addiction force someone to put a stake in something and then lose it all? There are several factors at play when it comes to dealing with the growing problem of addiction.

Cravings are a serious issue that torment numerous people fighting drug addiction, especially when they try to come off the addictive substance. Ironically, many people would have successfully attained long-term sobriety if cravings did not crop up with addiction. Apart from being considered as the major obstacles in recovery, cravings are also the root cause of relapse.

A complete recovery from addiction happens only when a person is free from cravings. Living a drug-free life without the need for constant monitoring against drug cravings can be difficult for a recovering individual, but a recent study published in the journal, Learning and Memory, has suggested that drug cravings can be effectively treated with vagus nerve stimulation (VNS). Under this therapy, patients are taught new behaviors that replace their old addictive behavior of seeking drugs.

Role of VNS in addiction recovery

In the University of Texas at Dallas study, the researchers revealed that the VNS therapy helped patients recover from the maladaptive behavior of drug taking. VNS is basically a surgical process wherein a device is implanted to a wire threaded along the vagus nerve, which travels up from the neck to the brain and connects with the area responsible for regulating mood. As small as a silver dollar, the device works like a pacemaker. It primarily works by sending a slight electric pulses through the vagus nerve, which further reaches the brain, thereby controlling cravings and urges.

The methodology is approved by the U.S. Food and Drug Administration (FDA) and is considered as a potential treatment for treatment-resistant depression, post-traumatic stress disorder (PTSD) and paralysis. The study further highlighted that VNS facilitates the "extinction learning" of drug seeking behaviors by reducing cravings and replacing the behavior associated with addiction with new ones. "Extinction of fearful memories and extinction of drugseeking memories relies on the same substrate in the brain. In our experiments, VNS facilitates both the extinction learning and reduces the relapse response as well," said Dr. Sven

Kroener of the University of Texas at Dallas.

A drug-free life is possible

Though addictive substances succeed in temporarily alleviating the emotional and physical pains of drug abusers, they have to eventually cope with the painful symptoms of substance abuse. Besides developing a number of physical and mental problems, many of these individuals also become self-destructive and suicidal.

Addiction to any substance can be life threatening. Only a comprehensive treatment program involving detoxification, medications, psychotherapies and other experiential therapies like yoga, meditation etc. can help an individual get sober. Moreover, a holistic recovery management plan is equally important to sustain the period of sobriety and manage cravings.

However, the extent to which health care practitioners can garner results in the treatment for drug addiction is dependent on the clinical characteristics of the patients that vary according to the type of drug abused as well as its quantity, duration, and the method of use (oral or intravenous).

Chapter 10:
Vagus Nerve Stimulation for Trauma, Chronic Fatigue, Obesity, and Fibromyalgia

Trauma

The body experiences other distressing signs of post-traumatic stress: tightness in the abdomen, a sinking sensation in the stomach, a familiar pain in the mouth, or a constant sense of fatigue. We now understand that as a part of the recovery process, we have to turn to the body. Thus, we have seen an increase in the use of meditation, mindfulness, tai chi, qigong, Feld ink circle, massage, craniosacral therapy, dietary therapy, and acupuncture for post-traumatic stress disorder.

Such mind-body treatments are helping us to be less passive, less aggressive, and less impulsive to stress. We're understanding the options we need to make us stay grounded and relaxed. We feel increasingly more in need of this. One way that mental-body treatments operate is by activating the vagus nerve. Awareness of how this nerve works offers a profound understanding of traumatic stress and promotes our healing capacity. The vagus nerve has, therefore, taken center stage in the treatment of trauma.

Moreover, mental-body treatments are successful as they require structural improvements in the autonomic nervous system as determined by the increase in vagus nerve activity. The vagus nerve reaches through the muscles of the nose, inner ear, chest, back, lungs, stomach, and intestines from the brainstem down. Mind-body treatments change how we relate to our surroundings by allowing us to try new breathing or activity patterns that communicate specifically with other parts of the body. Researchers also calculate the changes that exist in the vagus nerve, often referred to as the respiratory sinus arrhythmia by heart rate variability (HRV). HRV refers to the rhythmic heart rate oscillations that arise with the breath. It's a function of the intervals between beats in the heart. A higher variability in heart rate is associated with a better ability to withstand or rebound from stress.

Chronic Fatigue

If you find you are suffering from chronic fatigue, your vagus nerve may be the suspect, and that is good news. You can activate your vagus nerve regularly in hopes of getting out of this negative loop where you are too fatigued to get this nerve functioning properly, which then leads you to struggle further. Essentially, you need to figure out how to get yourself back into the proper parasympathetic state, and the fatigue will begin to go away on its own.

However, sometimes, the reason why you feel fatigued in general is that you are either finding yourself in constant sympathetic activation, even if only mildly, or you find you are teetering on the verge of a parasympathetic shutdown. Either of these situations could directly lead you to feel fatigued and unable to cope.

It's long been known that chronic fatigue syndrome can be triggered by viral infections, and that a non-stop immune response may result in devitalizing fatigue. For many years, experts in the medical field believed that it is a person's individual susceptibility that gives birth to the ecology for a particular disease state to take form. Regardless, many have thought that the vagus nerve plays a role in chronic fatigue syndrome, as well as a number of other common health problems. The scientist, Michael B. VanElzakker, in particular, argued that chronic fatigue syndrome is a result of the infection of the vagus nerve.

Every time an immune cell detects an infection, it releases cytokines that promote inflammation. These substances are detected by the vagus nerve receptors, which in turn signals the brain to activate fatigue, along with myalgia, fever, cold, flu, bacterial infection, and depression. According to VanElzakker, symptoms of chronic fatigue are the same as those of normal sickness, except they are triggered whenever a bacterium or virus infects the vagal ganglia. The cells activated by the intrusion can attack the vagus nerve by releasing cytokines and other substances that initiate sickness symptoms. This theory shows that the primary cause of chronic fatigue syndrome is the infection of the vagus nerve.

Obesity

The brain may relate how hungry or full you are, but at the end of the day, the vagus nerve is the part of the body that tells the stomach what the brain says. The brain functions as a sort of processor for the body, but if the vagus nerve is sending the wrong signals down to your stomach, you may find that you feel hungrier. You may find that the messages of having enough in your stomach never make it up to the brain or they are skewed in some way.

Because the vagus nerve makes up the gut-brain axis through which the stomach and the brain communicate, it can directly be implicated when something goes wrong. Whether something is failing to activate properly, or it realizes that your body needs more blood sugar, the vagus nerve may very well be at fault.

When it comes to obesity, it is often due to some sort of dysfunctional relationship with food. There are always circumstances in which a hormone leads to weight gain, but for the vast majority of people, that is not the case. Actually, when there is overeating and not enough exercise occurring, it can be a problem. As the years go on, the population becomes increasingly obese. This may be due to the fact that we do not have to be as active anymore. We do not have to run around to make sure we meet all of our needs because we don't have to hunt.

You do not have to make sure that you are able to fight off animals or are capable of defending your family to the same degree that you once did; and because of that, you may find that at the end of the day, you are growing complacent. You are busy with work, so you do not exercise. You are too busy, so you grab a pizza on the way home. You drive everywhere because it is easier. Suddenly, your caloric needs are actually much lower than they would be for a human out in the wild, having to hunt, grow food, and defend his or her home from that hungry bear desperate to get in.

Some people, after gaining weight, find that they just cannot lose it no matter how hard they try. These people may end up seeking weight loss surgery, which is invasive and entirely irreversible. When it is done, there is no turning back. However, studies have found that you can actually use the vagus nerve to aid in weight loss. In blocking the vagus nerve, the individual is much more likely to feel full for longer. This means the individual will not be overeating if the vagus nerve gets the wrong message.

In a clinical trial involving 233 people with BMIs of 35 or over, those who had the experimental generator activated lost roughly 8.5% more body weight over a year than their peers who did not get the shocks. Roughly half of the patients in this experimental group found that they lost up to 20% of their excess weight, while another 38% lost 25% of that excess weight. On the other hand, the patients who did not get the shocks during this time found that only 32.5% lost 20% of their weight, and only 23.4% lost 25%.

These results reveal that there is some degree of promise in using the vagus nerve to curb appetite to alleviate obesity without having to remove a portion of the stomach.

Fibromyalgia

There is still not much known about fibromyalgia, as the pain does not come from a specific cause or area in the body. Many researchers believe that with fibromyalgia, painful sensations are amplified due to the way the brain processes pain. A real reason is not fully known regarding this issue.

Sometimes the pain is triggered by a particular event, like an accident or surgery. Other times, there is no single experience, but the pain just seems to accumulate over time. There is no cure for fibromyalgia at this moment. However, there are interventions, both medical and nonmedical, that can help with subsiding the symptoms that come with it. Once again, our friend, the vagus nerve, is at play.

In a 2011, in an NIH study, the leading researchers suggested that vagus nerve stimulation may be a useful adjunct treatment for fibromyalgia patients. Further research is definitely needed, though. Many researchers feel that vagus nerve stimulation is effective in treating pain because it is able to negate a wide variety of factors that contribute to pain, like inflammation and the pain response.

There is still much that is up in the air about fibromyalgia. However, the results of such studies continue to suggest that the pain associated with it is significantly reduced with vagus nerve stimulation. Pain is often heightened when the body is stress. Since the vagus nerve can lower a person's stress through the sympathetic response, it is reasonable to believe that it can reduce or even eliminate pain associated with fibromyalgia.

Chapter 11:
Vagus Nerve Stimulation for Depression

D epression and anxiety are intricately linked. You probably don't need to know in great detail about depression since you're probably experiencing it. However, it is worthwhile to take the time to understand the biological underpinnings of it. This will make evaluating treatment options a lot easier. In addition to this, you'll also learn how the vagus nerve affects depression and can be used to improve your state of mind.

Your Brain on Depression

Just like the way anxiety is a perfectly normal and natural response in short doses, feelings of sadness and disappointment are similar. Sadness is simply the other side of the coin from happiness, and it is impossible to have one without the other. The issue arises when this balance is eroded, and a person begins to feel only one emotion predominantly.

As weird as it sounds, chronic and excessive happiness are harmful. We just don't see any cases of it because of our brain's inbuilt negativity bias. What we instead see pre-dominantly is a chronic state of excessive sadness, and this is what depression really is.

Depression was never really seen as a legitimate health concern for long periods of time. These days, the conversation around it is changing, thankfully, but there are still are significant roadblocks. Seeking therapy, for example, is still considered shameful in some cultures and men in particular face ridicule more often than not if they report themselves as being depressed in some parts of the world

(Koskie, 2018).

As a result, the data on depression is a bit skewed. In the United States, women are thought to be more likely to suffer depressive episodes. However, we don't know if this is simply because more women are willing to report depressive episodes than men. One can understand why men wouldn't want to concede any symptoms of perceived weakness since this is how we're brought up.

It is an experience I've undergone and struggled with massively. Following an accident, I intellectually understood that all the thoughts in my head were false and there were massive biological forces at work. I was the one in control, and I was the one causing these depressive episodes.

However, one cannot apply reasons when emotion strikes. The tidal wave of sadness and hopelessness that hit me left me devastated, despite all the scientific research and facts I had in my possession. CBT, as a therapeutic technique, helped immensely with this since it attacked the problem's biological root by focusing on building neural network forming habits.

Before we go into treatment options, though, let's take some time to take a look at the different types of depression. It is extremely relevant at this point because there are significant repercussions of untreated depression. Understand that in more serious cases, you should always seek professional help. Self-help techniques only go so far when it comes to depression, and this is why it is a bigger problem than anxiety. I'm not diminishing anxiety by any means but only trying to highlight just how huge a problem depression is.

Types of Depressive Disorders

Changing the language around depression is crucial. People who are depressed tend to associate their identities with it by using statements such as "I'm depressed." Thinking of it as a disorder helps dissociate from it. If you had a fever all of a sudden, you wouldn't blame yourself. You'd simply take your medicine and rest and eventually get over it. It sounds hard to think of depression in this manner, but over time, doing so will help you manage your situation better.

Persistent Depressive Disorder: This disorder is also called dysthymia and is present in around one percent of American adults (Koskie, 2018). Women are considered more susceptible, but I've already addressed how data reporting skews numbers. The condition itself refers to low-level depression that lasts for a long time, usually for two or three years.

Bipolar Disorder: This disorder is present in around 3% of Americans, with a whopping 83% of cases considered severe. The disorder manifests as a series of manic episodes where the patient appears to be overly energetic and has a lack of control over their actions. Major depression follows or precedes (or both) the manic episode.

Seasonal Affective Disorder (SAD): As the name suggests, seasonal changes bring about changes in mood. More often than not, the transition from summer to winter causes the condition due to the lack of sunlight. As a result, it is mostly reported in Northern European countries and places that experience significant swings between summer and winter temperatures.

Postpartum Depression: Despite the huge amount of literature dedicated to pregnancy, it is interesting that not enough has been written about postpartum depression. After all, 80% of new mothers experience this (Koskie, 2018). Hormonal changes and the stress of taking care of a new baby causes it. According to a study, close to 15% of new mothers are likely to experience a depressive episode within three months of childbirth (Koskie, 2018).

Psychotic Depression: Major depressive disorders may be accompanied by hallucinations and paranoia. This is when psychotic depression exists. Patients are usually admitted to a hospital when suffering from this disorder. Rather alarmingly, a study indicates that one in 13 people worldwide is likely to suffer from a psychotic depressive incident before the age of 75 (Koskie, 2018).

Major Depressive Disorder: This is the most commonly reported type of depressive disorder. This condition refers to a single instance of a depressive episode. Understand that sadness and depression are two completely different things. The World Health Organization (WHO) says that 300 million people worldwide suffer from depression, and it is the primary disability that exists currently.

Symptoms

The biggest and most obvious symptom of depression is a feeling of sadness that won't go away after a week or so. In addition to this, patients report a feeling of emptiness for this period of time. Depression is preceded by anxiety, and as a result, the symptoms of anxiety apply here as well.

Constant anxiety accompanied by feelings of restlessness is almost always a precursor to depression. Irritability and an inability to focus on the present are also symptoms. Constantly replaying past events and trying to correct them in some manner indicates depression. Patients at this point will have trouble controlling their tempers and will lash out at those around them. This is just an expression of the frustration they feel about their inability to make changes to situations they find themselves in.

As time goes on and anger dissipates, the patient starts moving away from the activities they used to engage in regularly. As this behavior intensifies, pretty much every thought or feeling that comes into their head is a negative one, and the constant pain becomes unbearable. Thus, the patient tends to disconnect from all emotions and tries to place themselves outside of any feelings. This is a close to impossible task since it isn't possible to be numb all the time.

Sensing the hopelessness of the situation, thoughts of suicide and other homicidal thoughts could follow. As you can see, there are various degrees of depression, and the symptoms vary as the condition gets worse. Physically, all of these mental symptoms manifest as oversleeping, insomnia, tircdness, constant aches and pains, irritability and weight changes, either loss or gain.

Is it possible to nip depression in the bud? The key to doing this is to understand the factors that increase the risk of depression.

Risk Factors

The primary risk factor is of depression genetic. If a person's family history shows cases of depression, they're more likely to suffer from it as well. Childhood traumatic experience such as sexual or physical abuse also increase the risk of becoming depressed. Chronic inflammation or diseases also increase the risk of depression.

Chronic inflammation is an extremely underrated cause of depression. When chronic inflammation has an extremely negative effect on the body, a person is likely to develop a negative state of mind. In younger people, low self-esteem is a major risk factor.

Prescription medication can cause depression

Some medicines inhibit the production of endorphins (the so-called "feel-good hormones") in the body, while others disrupt the digestive system by wiping out the probiotic gut flora. This leads to general irritability, and as a result, the mind-body connection suffers, and depression is the result. Lastly, constant alcohol or drug use only makes depression worse over the long term despite providing short-term relief.

Treatment

Just like with anxiety, the treatment for depression is a combination of medication and therapy. The prescription of medication depends on the severity of the patient's symptoms. More often than not, people who seek treatment for depression end up taking some medication. This is because we tend to take depression seriously only when it gets out of hand.

The World Health Organization states that less than 50% of people worldwide who suffer from depression seek treatment (Koskie, 2018). Studies have shown that relapse is possible after the treatment has been administered. In the case of therapy, relapse is possible for up to two years. Exact numbers aren't available here, thanks to the lack of a strict definition of which state of mind exactly qualifies as being depressed.

As a result, doctors generally conclude that a person who has suffered from a depressive episode once is extremely likely to relapse at some point. A special case is seasonal depression. Given that this condition arises primarily from a lack of natural light, light therapy is often prescribed. Natural spectrum lamps work just as regular light bulbs do, and these often relieve symptoms of SAD.

Consequences

Untreated depression has serious consequences, far more than anxiety and stress. Again, this isn't to minimize the latter conditions but is said more to highlight the seriousness of ignoring depression. For starters, chronic depression almost always results in drug or alcohol abuse of some kind.

Chronic inflammation is also one of the results of untreated depression, and leads to its own consequences, such as contracting autoimmune diseases and other untreatable diseases. While depression is not the cause of these diseases, their roots lie in its existence. Without depression, the odds of a person contracting chronic inflammation are pretty low after all.

Social isolation is almost always present when a person becomes depressed. You will learn more about this, but social disconnection and depression have strong biological links, and the degree of socialization a person is exposed to can directly affect their mental state.

Chapter 12:
Vagus Nerve Stimulation for PTSD

P ost-traumatic stress disorder is something that can be absolutely debilitating. Understanding PTSD and how it relates to the vagus nerve can help you figure out how best to deal with this trauma. It can help you develop the techniques you need to cope. We will address two exercises that can help with PTSD—using both deep-breathing and cold therapy to trigger the vagus nerve to alleviate the symptoms and side effects common to PTSD.

What is Post-Traumatic Stress Disorder?

Some people are suffering from post-traumatic stress disorder. When this happens, these individuals have repeated, persistent, and terrifying thoughts and flashbacks. They suffering from all of the anxiety of the instance that traumatized them: they may have repeated nightmares. They may find that they cannot focus or work. Even details that are hardly significant to the trauma at all, such as the weather or the sight of something they had seen just before the trauma trigger them, and they have flashbacks after being exposed.

Effectively, these people feel like ethe traumatic instance is reactivated over and over again without their input, and they are unable to do anything other than passively suffer through it. When this happens, they are miserable; it is hard to function when your body is constantly terrified of that traumatic ordeal happening again. You end up living your life trying to avoid things that may trigger the old feelings from resurfacing, but that is no way to live. You should not be living your life in fear of the past.

PTSD and the Vagus Nerve

Stop and consider the vagus nerve's role in response to trauma for a moment. When you are exposed to trauma, such as being attacked by someone or getting in a car accident, your body instantly goes into fight or flight mode. As you know, this is regulated by the vagus nerve, and it triggers the sympathetic nervous system.

This means that the trauma causes a suppression of the parasympathetic nervous system. This leads to an elevated heart rate and the individual being prepared to fight off the threat or run from it. The flight or fight response is considered to be a high activation of the sympathetic nervous system. On the other hand, during lower levels of activation, it is common to see a response known as freeze or faint. When this happens, the individual breathes shallowly and freezes up.

PTSD occurs when there is a lower activation of the sympathetic nervous system for a long period of time. The individual is constantly being exposed to stressors. Through triggering the vagus nerve and reminding the body to get out of fight-flight-freeze mode, you help mitigate the effects of PTSD. By reminding the body to reactivate the parasympathetic nervous system, you shut off all the negative responses. You can lessen the stress by regulating your body's ability to produce hormones to relax.

Diaphragmatic Breathing to Stimulate the Vagus Nerve

When you want to stimulate your nervous system, perhaps the easiest method is through diaphragmatic breathing. This can be done anywhere, and for the most part, can be incredibly discreet. All you need to do is breathe through your diaphragm to trigger the deep belly breaths that you will need if you wish to trigger the vagus nerve's activation.

Your diaphragm is the muscle in your lower belly underneath the lungs that contracts to allow you to draw air in and out of your lungs. People, especially women, tend to fall into the habit of breathing with the use of their chest instead of their diaphragm. Usually, due to vanity or wanting to suck in their stomach areas to appear thinner, this directly alters the way that you breathe.

When can trigger diaphragmatic breathing, however, you will find that you can ease also the sympathetic nervous system response. You can trigger the vagal activity that will help your body regulate itself. Any sort of deep breathing with your diaphragm will work. If you already have the knowledge how to do this, then make it a point to add it in during your day. If you are getting too stressed out, or you notice that your own PTSD symptoms seem to be flaring up, feeling like you are going to have flashbacks or that anxiety gnawing away at you, try to use your deep breathing. If you do not know how to breathe through your diaphragm, try the following:

1. Find somewhere quiet, so you can focus without distractions.

2. Place your right hand onto your stomach, right above your belly button

3. Place your left hand atop your heart.

4. Take in a deep breath and pay special attention to which hand is moving the most. If you notice that your right hand is the one that moves, you are already breathing with your diaphragm. If your left-hand moves more, you are breathing through your chest.

5. If you are breathing through your chest, take a deep breath, and focus on moving your belly as well. Practice this a few times while paying attention to how it feels.

With diaphragmatic breathing figured out, begin to utilize it in slow breathing exercises. You can use any breathing exercise that works for you, but one that works well is to breathe in and out for five seconds at a time.

You can do this with the following steps:

- Begin by inhaling through your nose slowly. Inhale as you slowly count to 5. If you cannot manage to fit that much oxygen into your body at one time, start with 4 seconds in. Pay attention to how the oxygen fills your lungs, expanding them.

- Hold the breath in your lungs for four seconds.

- Slowly begin to exhale, doing so for the 4 or 5 seconds that you inhaled as well.

- Repeat

Do the exercise for at least three or four minutes at a time. Some people prefer to fit this into their daily routine of meditations or yoga. No matter how you utilize it in your life, it can be useful in pulling the mind out of the fight or flight response.

Laughter to Stimulate the Vagus Nerve

Similarly to the way deep breathing can stimulate the vagus nerve, another commonly used tactic is to utilize deep laughter. When you were inhaling and exhaling, you were able to trigger the vagus nerve thanks to the way the breath moved through your body and your stomach expanded. When you are laughing at something or someone, you are moving your body in a very similar manner. This means that a good laughing session is actually going to trigger your vagus nerve, much like deep breathing did. This means that laughter may literally be the medicine that can best help you.

One of the best ways to trigger long-lasting laughter is finding a comedian that resonates with you. Find someone that you find has a similar sense of humor, and do not hesitate to watch them. In watching them and triggering the response of laughing, you will find that you can activate the vagus nerve, give yourself a workout, and have a good, mood-raising experience all by taking the time to laugh. Keep in mind that this cannot be fake laughing—you need to genuinely laugh those big belly laughs that everyone tries to get out of babies. Your laughing should engage your face, your chest, and your stomach, and the series of movements should be enough to activate the vagus nerve.

Chapter 13:
Vagus Nerve Hacking

T here are some methods of vagus nerve stimulation that you can't do yourself. Instead, you'll need to find a licensed professional. There are also methods of vagus nerve stimulation that aren't quiet exercises but are small lifestyle adjustments that can have big implications for your health. These will be divided into two parts: alternative therapies and lifestyle changes.

Massage Therapy

There are varieties of massage therapies, and just about all of them activate the vagus nerve in one way or another. Massage therapy doesn't just make you feel relaxed but it helps the muscles, bones, and even organs of the body to release pent up tensions. This release of tension brings the body out of the dangerous state and allows the vagus nerve to initiate the healing processes that are impossible when the muscles and joints are tensed for action.

Chronic tension in the muscles can even impact your skeletal structure. Massage therapy has been found to realign the bone structure, which improves blood circulation, nerve function (of all kinds) and even takes the pressure off the spinal cord. Massaging of the feet has been linked to a lowering of heart rate and blood pressure, which in return takes the pressure off the vagus nerve.

Reflexology

Reflexology therapy has its origins in traditional Chinese medicine, but in recent years, it has spread all over the world as its positive benefits are becoming commonly known. The technique behind reflexology is to activate certain pressure points in the feet, which have beneficial results throughout the body. While the vagus nerve itself doesn't extend to the feet, stimulating the pressure points in the feet can do a lot to relax the body and take it out of its dangerous state, allowing the vagus nerve to assume its role as the body's healer in the state of safety. It has also been linked to improved circulation, which does directly stimulate the vagus nerve.

Acupuncture

Like reflexology, acupuncture also comes to us from traditional Chinese medicine. While this healing technique is still being discovered by the West, it's been practiced in almost the exact same way in China and East Asia for thousands of years. Some of the first medical books ever written in any language are books on acupuncture.

This technique stimulates certain pressure points throughout the body, allowing the body to relax and release tension. The Chinese explain this as improving the flow of energy throughout the body. When the energy flow is clogged up, the body falls prey to a number of illnesses. Acupuncture is designed to open up the energy pathways in the body to keep vital energy circulating in a healthy way.

This might sound new age to a Western mind, but from a holistic medical perspective, it actually makes a great deal of sense. In modern medical speak, we think of acupuncture as stimulating certain nerves, with the understanding that those nerves are connected to multiple organs in the body. An acupuncture nerve above the knee or the shoulder, for example, may indeed ignite neural signals that make their way back to the digestive tract, the brain, or the heart, and therefore contribute to whole-body wellness.

Lifestyle and Diet Adjustments

Probiotics

Believe it or not, there are also bacteria that are bad good for you. In fact, there is a whole culture of bacteria that lives in your gut that is not only good but necessary for healthy digestive function. When the health of the gut microbiome is compromised, it can have consequences for the entire body. The gut microbiome is continuously sending signals from the gut to the brain, which is the primary way the brain monitors and regulates healthy digestive function. And guess which nerve carries those signals? You guessed it - the vagus nerve. In fact, a significant portion of the vagus nerve is connected to the gut and its microbiome. If the gut microbiome is compromised, it can shut down the entire nerve.

Probiotics are good bacteria. Consuming probiotics helps to keep our guts (and our vagus nerve) healthy, happy, and fully functional. Probiotics are primarily found in fermented foods. Kefir, kimchi, kombucha, tempeh, miso, sauerkraut, sourdough, natto, and even beer are all examples of fermented foods that are chock full of healthy probiotics that are great for improving and maintaining gut health.

Healthy Fats

There are three ways that the body gains energy from food: carbohydrates, fats, and proteins. These are called macronutrients, and you must consume at least one of the three every day for your cells to survive. While most diets are high in carbs and proteins, the best diet for the vagus nerve (believe it or not) is a high-fat diet.

However, a "high fat" diet implies a "low carb" diet. The reason that healthy fats are better than carbs as the body's main energy source is that carbs are pure energy, while fats contain other vitamins, nutrients, and chemicals called ketones, which initiate healing processes at the cellular level. A high fat, low carb diet is the best for a healthy digestive tract and will therefore relieve a great deal of stress from the vagus nerve, which is constantly at work to keep your digestion running smoothly and healthily.

Laughter and Positive Social Interactions

A healthy social life also stimulates the vagus nerve. Laughter is both a physical and psychological stimulator for the vagus nerve, as this is yet another autonomic reflex regulated by the vagus nerve. Positive social interactions do an amazing job in the brain to make the body feel safe, secure and protected. Going long periods of time without positive social interactions can definitely throw the body into a defensive state, which in turn shuts down the vagus nerve.

During positive social engagement, these muscles actual make numerous involuntary movements that signal safety and positive communication to the other person. Sending and receiving these signals, again, stimulates the vagus nerve and causes the body to initiate a number of healing processes. More importantly, these signals cannot be sent or received via remote communication, even through video communication. Therefore, in order to stimulate the vagus nerve, positive social interactions must happen in real life, rather than over the phone or the internet.

Sleep on your Right Side

Sounds weird, but it's actually been found to work. Why? Remember that your heart isn't located in the center of your chest. In fact, it's actually positioned slightly to the left. Sleeping on the left side can be a hassle for the cardiovascular muscles when you sleep, which puts stress on your heart and decreases heart rate variability. Sleeping on the right, on the other hand, gives your heart the maximum amount of space (even more than laying on your back), which improves heart rate variability and subsequently stimulates the vagus nerve and improves vagal tone.

Supplements

Fish Oil

Fish oil supplements contain two chemicals called EPA and DHA. These two chemicals have both been shown to improve heart rate variability, lower the heart rate, and subsequently improve vagal tone. Just one fish oil supplement daily is enough to improve functionality in the heart and stimulation the vagus nerve.

Oxytocin

Oxytocin is another chemical that has been found to stimulate activity in the vagus nerve. Specifically, oxytocin allows the brain to relax and stimulates healthy digestive activity. Oxytocin can be taken as a supplement. Just one supplement daily is enough to stimulate activity in the vagus nerve.

Zinc

Zinc is a very rampant mineral found in a number of different fruits and veggies. Unfortunately, most people don't get nearly enough plants in their diets, and subsequently, don't get enough of this healing mineral. Zinc alone has been found to stimulate the vagus nerve, and it can be taken as a supplement for the optimal improvement of vagus nerve activity. However, eating a plant-based diet that consists of a variety of fruits and vegetables will not only get you enough natural zinc to keep your vagus nerve happy, but it will also flood your body with a number of other vitamins and nutrients that improve gut and organ health.

Serotonin

Serotonin is a chemical that is made in the brain to regulates mood. Serotonin is produced naturally when you are engaged in certain activities that bring you pleasure, including exercises, eating a delicious meal, having sex, or hanging out with friends. However, long periods of anxiety, depression, or drug abuse can cause a serotonin deficiency in the brain, which, in turn, throws the body into a dangerous state and compromises the vagus nerve. If you've experienced severe anxiety, depression, or are recovering from drug addiction, you may want to consider taking serotonin supplements to help the body remain relaxed and in a state of safety until the vagus nerve can do its healing work. Serotonin supplements can be purchased over the counter and have fewer negative side effects than antidepressants or other anxiety medications.

Fiber

Fiber is a nutrient found primarily in plant-based foods. Fiber acts as a gut cleaner, flushing out toxins that have built up in the intestines. When we don't get enough fiber in our diets, certain toxic materials can build up over time and put stress on the gut microbiome, which, in turn, compromises the vagus nerve. A plant-based diet rich in whole fruits and vegetables will naturally get you enough of it to keep your gut (and your vagus nerve) happy and healthy. You can also take fiber as a supplement or even sprinkle it over your food as a powder.

Sun Exposure

Simply getting sun on your skin can stimulate the vagus nerve. Believe it or not, the body is actually designed to absorb a number of vitamins and nutrients (most notably vitamin D) directly from the sun. Some of these vitamins initiate beneficial chemical reactions in the brain and central nervous system. Remember that the vagus nerve is one of the biggest nerves in the central nervous system, so activation of the central nervous system also stimulates the vagus nerve.

Chapter 14:
Vagus Nerve Exercises

E xercise and physical movement challenge you and give you a sense of accomplishment, which directly opposes the miserable feeling that depression causes. In case of anxiety is your issue, exercise gives you an opportunity to vent your frustration at something. Exercise also releases endorphins in your system and helps you feel better. All in all, there is no downside to exercise, and you should aim to make it a part of your daily routine.

Diaphragmatic Breathing

Most people will inhale up to 14 times per minute and in doing so, they have superficial breathing. When you become more self-aware of your breathing rate, you are able to lower the amount to an ideal breathing rate of 6 inhales per minute. This forces your body to practice deeper breathing techniques and fill your lungs to capacity with each breath. It's incredibly easy to practice this routine wherever you may be. I'm practicing it right now as I type!

This type of breathing exercise especially helps to trigger the vagus nerve and turns on its full activation as it is telling the brain that it is now necessary to calm down, even though the nerve itself has not been given that particular instruction directly. In this way, the mechanism is the same as when you close your eyes and tap your eyelids gently. Your brain will perceive each tap as a spark of light shining through.

When we breathe in deeper breaths, we are making use of the lower part of our chests and moving the diaphragm in such a way that it will promote relaxation.

The Power of Stretching

Stretching is used to help naturally stimulate the body and make movement simple. There is a lot you can get out of this. Most people don't realize that they're not only releasing tension within the muscles when they stretch, but they're also focusing their breathing; so it's simple and yet very useful.

A lot of people don't stretch enough, so tension sits there. But a way to naturally start up the parasympathetic nervous system and activate the vagus nerve is to do this: sit down and stretch out your body to promote relaxation and wellness, and from there, stretching will stimulate your entire body.

Try touching your toes, stretching your arms behind your head, pushing them up, holding your arms in the air, or even just moving towards your foot will help with this. There is a lot of benefit to be had. You'll be shocked and amazed, and most of all, you'll be quite happy with the power of this small exercise. You'll feel invigorated and ready for whatever come in the future.

Consider stretching right before you begin your day or at the end of the evening, and see how it helps you feel during the day. You'll feel your vagus nerve stimulated almost immediately.

Weight Training

Weight training might seem weird to stimulate the vagus nerve, but it does work. That's because, when you lift weights, it changes the speed of the body. Plus, through the power of repetition, you get your body to relax. A lot of people thinks that lifting weights is only for big, burly people, but that isn't the case.

Ever just doing a few sets of curls will change the way your body feels. Many people think they need to start with a heavyweight right away, but that isn't the case either.

HIIT Workouts

HIIT, or High-Intensity Interval Training, is a form of workout that require a lot in a minimal period. Sometimes, it involves sprinting; other times, it can be push-ups, sit-ups, or other exercises. The main goal is to do a lot in a short time through spurts.

These spurts cause vagus nerve stimulation. The vagus nerve is usually not stimulated if you're always stressed out. Still, the periods of stress and then relaxation kick the vagus nerve into gear, helping it activate whenever needed.

HIIT workouts are also exceptional because they are straightforward. No matter what you do, you'll feel the difference immediately.

Walking

Walking is an excellent option if you're not going to the gym or don't want to spend time doing HIIT or yoga. Walking is an excellent habit because it stimulates your body and helps with physical fitness and wellness. Your vagus nerve will get stimulated by walking, especially if you live a sedentary lifestyle.

I think walking for 30 minutes a day is ideal, especially if you're unable to do it more. Sometimes, pacing while on breaks is a great way to do it. In any case, walking improves your health and wellness. To help with your physical fitness, walking is a good start, especially if you're not otherwise active.

Jogging is also another good one because that helps with deep breathing. A lot of people, when they start, will get into the habit of breathing in short breaths, but that won't work here. This can make it hard to run, and you might pass out. With jogging, you want to make sure that you're breathing in a slow, deep, and even manner, and focus on this. This will help with your vagus nerve and get you into the habit of breathing deeply. You can also do some running, but it's more high-intensity, and it might be harder to engage in deep breathing.

Jumping

Jumping is another great form of cardio, and your vagus nerve will love it. Jumping jacks, burpees, and other jumping exercises are useful in improving circulation, which can help with blood pressure and your vagal tone.

When you jump, be mindful of your breathing. Try to do it with a deep breath; you'll notice it's a much harder workout, and you'll feel the difference. It increases blood flow, blood pressure, and heart rate as well. Your vagus nerve will thank you for this, and you'll be able to improve your health and wellness.

Yoga

There are not a lot of studies on the effects of yoga on the vagus nerve, but the ones that have been conducted suggest that yoga does increase vagus nerve activity. For instance, a 12-week yoga intervention was found to be more beneficial in terms of mood improvement than walking exercises. A study conducted on the effects of yoga on mood and anxiety found an increase in thalamic GABA levels, which are linked to decreased anxiety and improved mood.

Today, many consider yoga as an effective way to regulate the functioning of the vagus nerve. To practitioners, the goal of yoga in relation to the vagus nerve is to become increasingly flexible. Its main aim is to help people suffering from severe stress and trauma become skilled in switching between the parasympathetic and the sympathetic nervous system with less difficulty. Overall, yoga has been found to be good for improving overall physical and mental health, although more studies need to be conducted on its impact on vagal function.

Aerobics

Aerobics is another higher-intensity exercise, but some variants aren't as extensive or intensive as others. Zumba tends to be on the more intensive side, and there are different classes to try. However, there are other aerobic exercises, such as water aerobics, weight training, cycling, and even some types of yoga.

All of these, when combined, are wonderful for vagus nerve stimulation and great for the body. You'll be amazed at how helpful this can be for the body and how you can improve your vagus nerve. They encourage you to breathe, which promotes deeper breathing and, thereby, vagus nerve stimulation.

Swim It Out!

Swimming is a great aerobic exercise according to most experts, and if you're not a fan of jogging or running, or weight training, swimming is a good alternative. It helps in many ways. For starters, you're submerging your head, which stimulates the mammalian diving reflex, which includes your vagus nerve. It also pushes you to control your breathing as you move. You need to hold your breath but also walk through the water. As such, it is a combination of both techniques which provides correct vagus nerve stimulation. Plus, we all know that swimming improves bodily movement because you're moving about and encouraging blood flow too. You'll notice that as you begin, it's hard to do, but over time, you'll get better. It's a beautiful form of cardio, and it's ideal for properly stimulating the vagus nerve.

Dancing

Dancing is an excellent form of self-expression. Even if you're silly, it can help you feel much better about yourself. Dancing enables you to improve your physical fitness, gets the blood flow moving, and helps you stay active and fun.

There are so many different kinds of dance classes these days. You can do Zumba or other forms like ballroom. Some people even like ballet because it requires muscle control that can stimulate the vagus nerve. They're all fun to do, and they encourage you to move, control your breathing, and let you express yourself.

Even ethnic or interpretive dancing can help. And if it can make you laugh, it will naturally stimulates the vagus nerve in a fun way. All in all, dancing is excellent and lets you feel good about yourself. Consider dancing when you want to express yourself and feel good.

When it comes to stimulating the vagus nerve, these are all practical activities that boost the vagus nerve. Your vagus nerve is vital because it lets you relax the body and helps curb inflammation. But, while these exercises are great for stimulating it, they also get the body moving, which increases the vagal tone. They help offset obesity, diabetes, and other conditions related to weight.

High-Intensity Interval Sprinting

High-intensity interval sprinting stimulates the vagus nerve by waking up the heart and lungs. Doing this one to two times a week will provide the necessary stimulation to the nerve. To do this exercise, run as fast as you possibly can for 30 seconds and then walk for two minutes. This is one cycle. Repeat it for 10 minutes to get a full workout.

Cardio Machines

Treadmills or other walking machines at the gym are great if you don't have a pleasant place to walk outdoors. Especially for those who are living in cold climates, taking advantage of a treadmill at the gym or even investing in one for your home is an excellent way to keep you walking every day, indoors or out.

Jump Rope

Did you ever jump or skip rope as a child? This childhood game is a great way to get your heart beating and your lungs expanding with fresh air. Find a basic child's jump rope and jump for two to five minutes a day to stimulate the vagus nerve. This can be done indoors (of course), but if you can, try to do it outside to get the extra benefits of fresh air and sun exposure.

Resistance Training

Otherwise known as weightlifting, this does more than just grow the muscles in your arms and legs. It also stimulates the cardiovascular system and speeds up metabolism, which, in turn, stimulates the vagus nerve. There are many types of resistance training to explore with your trainer or a savvy friend.

Chapter 15:
Meditation for Vagus Nerve Activation

O ne of the essential ways of activating the vagus nerve is through meditation. Meditation can be used by anyone, even those who do not attend classes. As compared to tai-chi and yoga, which seem to be complex, meditation is a simple approach that involves visualization. The practitioner has to visualize a certain environment that promotes calmness. The main aim of meditation is to calm down the sympathetic action and activate the parasympathetic action of the vagus nerve. If you are capable of sending a signal to the brain that will initiate the actions of the parasympathetic nervous system, you will be in the best position to move on with your life.

To benefit from meditation, you need to choose the right type as but only a few are effective in calming down nerves and boosting vagus nerve action. Some of the meditation techniques used to activate the vagus nerve include:

Mindfulness Meditation: In this type, the aim is to distract the mind from the thoughts that cause anxiety. When you practice mindfulness meditation, the focus is on yourself. You only think about yourself, your body, and your environment. If you want to enjoy the fruits of mindful meditation, you need to observe the rules. First, during mindfulness, a person may discover some frustrating facts about themselves. In mindful meditation, you allow yourself to visualize yourself in a way that you have never done before. One of the most important rules is being non-judgmental. In other words, you are not permitted to judge yourself after observing your thoughts or feelings. You are required to embrace the truth about yourself. This action in itself promotes a calming of nerves.

Some people who suffer from depression only experience nervousness due to the fear of being judged. However, if you can learn to accept your flaws through mindfulness meditation, you will not be shaken by anything. Mindfulness meditation teaches you to stand strong and believe in yourself no matter what the world may say. This is the attitude you need to overcome anxiety and depression. This attitude also promotes the parasympathetic activities of the vagus nerve.

Focused Meditation: Focused meditation is a type where the practitioner focuses their thoughts on a single object. You can choose any object in a room – a chair or a wall. Focused meditation needs intense concentration. When performing focused meditation, you can't release your eyes from the object. Use your mind to describe its different aspects. Think about its design, colors, shape, make, or any other feature. Think about factors that make it special, for example, how it holds weight. This type of meditation is only intended to help you reduce the tension in your mind. After reducing the tension, the body can slowly reduce the sympathetic actions that are leading to anxiety.

Peace, Love, and Kindness Meditation: This is the ideal type of meditation for individuals looking to activate the vagus nerve. The fact that a person may be experiencing anxiety or depression means they need an activity that will lead to the calming down of nerves. There is no better activity than peace, love, and kindness meditation.

You visualize yourself as a center of peace, love, and kindness to the world. In your mind, you visualize a world without violence or hatred where you are the main source of peace, love, and kindness. You visualize yourself extending kindness to people who need it. You stand out as someone who embraces the weak. In your routines, you provide peace and kindness to people who are close to you and try to show them that the world can be a better place. You freely gift people who need help on the streets. You may also visit your enemies and extend a hand of forgiveness. Create a perfect world in your visualization, and just indulge in that peaceful world for a few minutes. When you are done with your meditation, you will be in the right place to let go of all your fears and anxiety. This calming effect activates the vagus nerve, allowing you to live a normal life again.

Simple Step by Step Guide to Meditation

Step1: Prepare the meditation room and tools

For meditation to be successful, you must find a quiet location without interruptions. You can meditate in your bedroom or in an open space. It is important that the meditation location have plenty of fresh air and allows you to enjoy peace during meditation. You will also need a meditation mat or a right-back chair. You may need some meditation music, but it is not compulsory.

Step 2: Position yourself for meditation

Before you start your meditation, ensure you have enough time to complete the session. Switch off your cell phone and only use your watch to set a reminder for timing purposes. Place yourself on the mat in a sitting posture with your legs right in front. Sit in an upright position and allow yourself to freely breathe in the fresh air. If you are using a chair, ensure your back is aligned parallel to the straight back of the chair. This allows your back to be in an upright position, which is perfect for free breathing.

Step 3: Prepare your mind for meditation

You now need to activate your concentration. The easiest way to start concentrating is by focusing on your breathing for about 5 minutes. Do not try controlling how you breathe. Just focus your thoughts and feel how the air goes in and comes out. This will raise your awareness of the environment and allow you to concentrate on the moment.

Step 4: Get into visualization

Once your mind has been prepared for the process, get deep into visualization. You can do this with any type of meditation. You start by preparing your room, positioning yourself, and preparing your mind. Once you are ready, you now focus your mind on whatever it is that the meditation technique requires. For instance, in focused meditation, you may open your eyes and choose to focus on the ceiling in the room. If you know that you'll be doing focused meditation, ensure there is something to focus on in the room. If you are performing peace, love, and kindness meditation, you have to close your eyes and create images in your head. You have to start visualizing your activities as an ambassador for peace to those who need it. It is much simpler if you close your eyes and only focus on the meditation for a given period of time.

Conclusion

Every time we discover something new about the body, we are left wondering at the amazing feats it is capable of, from controlling the immune system to the brain processing information. The body is truly a magnificent system, and each of its parts is an important and fascinating component of that system.

But that does not mean that the body can do everything on its own. We have to make sure we are helping the body function smoothly. Exercising and eating healthy are often repeated topics in healthcare. There is a reason for that repetition. They are important aspects of living and taking care of ourselves.

Certain components of the body require their own special care along with physical exercise and a good diet. For example, the brain needs to feel positive emotions be filled with mental exercises. The same goes for the vagus nerve.

For a long time, the scientific and medical communities never thought to examine the vagus nerve and its complex connections to the nervous system and the rest of the body. When they eventually did uncover its functions, they were surprised at the extent to which the vagus nerve influences the body. As with any new discovery, there was a mad scramble to figure out all the secrets of the vagus nerve and how you should take care of it.

Which eventually brings us to this book. You now have a compendium of knowledge in your hands about the vagus nerve, its influence on the body. Knowing more about the vagus nerve, you are one step closer not only to being aware of its powerful influences but also how you can take care of it.

It is up to you to focus on reducing inflammation in the body, lowering its levels of stress, and using proper routines to improve the conditions of your vagus nerve. It is your responsibility to see that yet another important component of the body is functioning properly.

Our brain alone contains about 100 billion neurons (Shulman, 2019). Yet, as amazing as the brain is, it can't function properly without help from the nervous system.

The vagus nerve isn't the only nerve in the body, but it's undoubtedly the longest. The vagus nerve is the thread that binds all of our inner organs together, facilitating a vast network of connections that run throughout the entire body. Directly or indirectly, everything that happens in the body is connected to the vagus nerve. It's the spark of life that keeps our organs working and our brain functioning. If this nerve can't do its job, then nothing in the body can function the way that it normally should.

As long as the vagus nerve is defensive and tense, it cannot regulate the organs homeostatically. The healing processes happening in a state of safety are disrupted or delayed. The digestive functions are chemically disturbed, and the health of the gut microbiome is compromised.

All the stimulating exercises, techniques, and procedures that facilitate vagus nerve function are designed with one primary goal—bringing the vagus nerve back into a state of safety. Everyone's brain is different, and not all of these healing techniques will work for you. Some will want to do them every day, while others you may only do them every week or even every month.

You may be someone who enjoys physical or medical interventions, and you may prefer physical exercises and diet changes. You may be prefer psychological interventions and opt for meditations and social engagement. The point is there is a way for everyone.

www.ingramcontent.com/pod-product-compliance
Lightning Source LLC
Chambersburg PA
CBHW060319030426
42336CB00011B/1122